THE
ART
AND
SCIENCE
OF
CONNECTION

THE
ART
AND
SCIENCE
OF
CONNECTION

Why Social Health Is the Missing Key
to Living Longer, Healthier, and Happier

KASLEY KILLAM, MPH

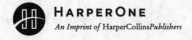

HarperOne
An Imprint of HarperCollinsPublishers

THE ART AND SCIENCE OF CONNECTION. Copyright © 2024 by Kasley Killam. All rights reserved. Printed in the United States of America. No part of this book may be used or reproduced in any manner whatsoever without written permission except in the case of brief quotations embodied in critical articles and reviews. For information, address HarperCollins Publishers, 195 Broadway, New York, NY 10007.

HarperCollins books may be purchased for educational, business, or sales promotional use. For information, please email the Special Markets Department at SPsales@harpercollins.com.

FIRST EDITION

Designed by Michele Cameron
Part opener art © Shutterstock

Library of Congress Cataloging-in-Publication Data has been applied for.

ISBN 978-0-06-328911-6

24 25 26 27 28 LBC 5 4 3 2 1

For Marcus, Mum, Kara, and Zac,
my unwavering sources of social health

Contents

Author's Note

The stories in this book are all true as told to me or experienced by me. In several cases, I changed names and certain details to protect people's privacy or merged stories to further anonymize, and some quotes have been edited for clarity. I'm grateful to everyone who trusted me with their perspectives; my favorite part of writing this book was connecting with you.

Communicating scientific findings in ways that are accurate, interesting, and useful is an art. The information in this book has been carefully researched, and all efforts have been made to ensure accuracy. The book picks up where the data leaves off with insights from experts and everyday people. I hope this makes for an enjoyable read that is both rooted in evidence and blossoming through lived experiences.

Introduction

The Future of Health Is Social

What do you do to be healthy?

Let's say you follow the advice of doctors, health blogs, and wellness influencers perfectly. You walk ten thousand steps per day. You get eight hours of quality sleep at night. You eat plenty of fresh vegetables and avoid processed foods. You work through challenges with a therapist. You meditate and take hot baths for self-care.

Your physical and mental health improve as a result—but only up to a point.

The problem with traditional health advice is that it overlooks one of the most important ingredients: human connection.

You can't be fully healthy if you don't have a name to write down as your emergency contact. If you don't see family except for a few hours over the holidays. If you lack close friends to share experiences with. Or if you don't have enough alone time to reconnect with yourself.

You value your romantic and platonic relationships, but do you know they determine how long you live? When you spend time with family or friends, invite a coworker to lunch, or strike up a conversation with a neighbor, do you realize the interaction influences whether or not you—and they—will develop heart disease, diabetes, depression, or dementia?[1]

Health is not only physical or mental. Health is also social.

Social health is the aspect of overall health and well-being that comes from connection—and it is vastly underappreciated. Whereas physical health is about your body and mental health is about your mind, social health is about your relationships. As we will explore in part I, being socially healthy requires cultivating bonds with family, friends, and the people around you, belonging to communities, and feeling supported, valued, and loved, in the amounts and ways that feel nourishing to you.

Decades of research have proven that connection is as essential as food and water, but this knowledge hasn't yet made its way into the mainstream understanding of health—and without it, we're suffering.

Today, many people show signs of social health in decline. Over the past thirty years, the percentage of Americans with ten or more close friends dropped by 20 percent.[2] Over the past twenty years, the amount of time people spent alone increased by an average of twenty-four hours per month.[3] Over the past ten years, participation in communities, such as book clubs, sports leagues, and neighborhood associations, fell by nearly 20 percent.[4] And according to a national survey in 2019, around half of adults in the US felt as if no one knew them well.[5]

Researchers have documented similar trends in other countries. According to Gallup, 330 million adults around the globe endure weeks at a time without speaking to a single family member or friend, and 20 percent of all adults worldwide don't have *anyone* they can reach out to for help.[6] These statistics stun even me, who reads statistics like these for a living.

This lack of connection is dangerous, increasing people's risk of stroke by 32 percent, their risk of dementia by 50 percent, and their risk of early death by 29 percent.[7]

But it's not just disconnection that takes a toll; an overwhelming amount of connection or unfulfilling connection does, too. Whether introverts drained by too many social obligations, extroverts spread too thin, teenagers overwhelmed by social media, or communities enmeshed in conflict, many people's social scales are off-balance. Meanwhile, hate crimes have surged,[8] polarization has escalated,[9] and people's sense of trust in one another is strained at best.[10]

This amounts to nothing short of a public health emergency. As we will explore in chapter 10, leaders around the world are beginning to mount a response, from governments in the UK and Japan appointing ministers for loneliness to the World Health Organization establishing a global Commission on Social Connection.

But what does this mean for you? What can *you* do in your everyday life to connect meaningfully with the people around you and live a longer, healthier, and happier life as a result?

I've spent over a decade answering that question. This book reveals exactly what I've learned, presenting new vocabulary for how to think and talk about the importance of connection with family, friends, spouses, coworkers, neighbors, and other social ties, as well as specific strategies to be more socially healthy.

DISCOVERING THE MISSING KEY

When I was growing up, the social world around me was complicated. At home, I felt loved and supported by my parents and siblings, but there were feuds, divorces, and estrangements that fractured both my nuclear and extended families irreparably. At school, I was confident in myself and had plenty of friends, yet I never felt that I fully fit in, and I was dismayed by the meanness I observed between cliques. Later, as an adult at work, I navigated being an introvert in a professional culture that rewards extroversion. Over the years, I moved multiple times to different cities, each time needing to figure out how to build a community from scratch while staying in touch with loved ones far away.

By the time I was in my early twenties, I was convinced that all these pieces fit together somehow, but how? I sensed that I was struggling with something, but what? I didn't even have the language to describe what was missing from my life—let alone the tools to fix it.

So, as a social scientist, I turned to the data for an answer. I devoured every academic paper I could find related to human connection, attended conferences to learn from leading researchers, and sought out opportunities such as working at the University of Pennsylvania's Positive Psychology Center and spending a summer as a visiting scholar with the Mind & Life Institute. I learned that prosocial behaviors—actions that connect us to others, such as gratitude, kindness, and empathy—rewire our brains and change the physiological functioning of our bodies. I learned that people not only are happier but also live longer when they have good relationships.

The stakes were higher than I had originally suspected. To live long and to live well, the data showed, we need love.

But I still couldn't put a finger on what all this really meant. It seemed that researchers were getting at a common theme from their different silos, but there was not a satisfying overarching narrative or clear path forward for everyday people like you and me going about our lives.

Then, in 2013, I received a grant from Stanford University to develop a campaign and mobile app to help people deepen their relationships—and that's when I found it. While gathering evidence for the project, I discovered the solution to the puzzle. The unifying theme. The language that captured what I was yearning for in life.

Social health.

In the early 1970s, a scholar at Southern Illinois University named Robert D. Russell published a paper titled "Social Health: An Attempt to Clarify This Dimension of Well-Being." He had noticed that the World Health Organization defined health as "a state of complete physical, mental and social well-being" but that no one had really developed the third component. Russell conducted surveys and interviews to arrive at a definition: social health, he wrote, is the "dimension of an individual's well-being that concerns how he gets along with other people, how other people react to him and how he interacts with social institutions and societal mores."

Everything clicked when I read this for the first time. "That's it!" I thought. "Now I just need to learn everything I can about social health and I'll be set."

Except there was almost nothing else available. I scoured the library and searched online, in academic journals and popular media. There was no shortage of information on related concepts, like social connectedness and even social well-being, but social health had a different—and crucial—connotation. Russell had passed away in 2005, and aside from a few mentions here and there, no one I could find had elaborated on his definition in a robust, meaningful way. Outside of academia, social health was glaringly absent from public discourse. (As I write this ten years later, there's still not even a Wikipedia page about social health.)

I was baffled. In the months and years that followed, I couldn't stop thinking about social health. To me, the term perfectly captured what I knew from science and personal experience to be true—that not just happiness, but also *health*, is inextricably linked to connection. I liked that it naturally extended the language that I and most people were already familiar with—building on physical and mental health with social health.

Yet it had been buried in academia for decades. I wondered: Had the idea of social health not made it into the mainstream because it didn't resonate with anyone other than me? Or because it had simply gone unnoticed—its potential underappreciated and waiting to be realized?

It was possible, I hypothesized, that social health just needed a good publicist.

Moreover, it needed a framework—a tangible approach for people to strengthen social health as we do physical and mental health. Since I couldn't find one, I was going to have to make one.

Over the next decade, I set out to do exactly that. First, I tested my hypothesis by using the term in conversations with friends and colleagues, writing articles about it for publications like *Scientific American* and *Psychology Today*, and giving talks about it for organizations across sectors and communities around the world.

People's reactions and feedback affirmed that the term *social health* resonated with more than just me. When I started spreading the message publicly, I felt like a soloist. I was stunned and delighted the first few times I heard or read someone else casually mention social health in conversation or in writing, as part of their normal vocabulary. Today, people in and out of my circles use it all the time, and there is a rapidly growing global choir that gets louder by the day.

Emboldened by the spreading of the term, I turned my attention to developing a methodology. I knew the real test of an idea isn't in a laboratory or dataset; it's in real life. So I started where I lived at the time, in San Francisco. I organized a public gathering and invited local leaders to speak about what they were hearing and seeing on the ground—learning that many older adults felt isolated and many teenagers were craving offline connection. At another event, I brought together younger and older community members for an afternoon of conversation across ages, which resulted in intergenerational friendships that continue to this day—showing me how easy it could be to spark connection. I joined the board of a local nonprofit that built community among older adults—seeing firsthand how people who went from isolated to connected experienced better health outcomes as a result.

Increasingly, I read news headlines about a rise in loneliness, which added fuel to the fire of my determination; this was a profound need in the world that I believed social health could help.

So, in 2019, I took a leap of faith by quitting my job at Verily, the health-tech spin-off of Google, to focus on social health full-time. I joined the Harvard T.H. Chan School of Public Health as a graduate student, where I gained perspective on the value of seeing individuals' health—whether physical, mental, or social—as not only influenced by their actions but also inseparable from the world around them. I learned which tools in the public health tool belt have advanced our collective understanding and improved humanity's health throughout history, and I studied how to use those to prevent loneliness and promote connection.

After graduating, I began advising and partnering with organizations to integrate these lessons into products, services, and campaigns. I also founded a nonprofit called Social Health Labs. My team and I launched a microgrant program to fund individual community builders in neighborhoods across the US—proving that truly anyone can build relationships locally with a little support and a lot of enthusiasm. We convened experts across industries and thousands of members of the public around the world in a series of conversations—uncovering innovative ways to reduce loneliness and identifying opportunities to strengthen social health throughout society.

With that, I had collected the remaining pieces of the puzzle and finally figured out how to fit them together.

Now I'm handing these insights over to you.

YOUR ROAD MAP FOR SOCIAL HEALTH

Unlike physical and mental health, social health as an idea and approach has not been developed in a practical way—until now.

In the following pages, I share what I have learned from over a decade of studying, practicing, and refining social health in my own life, with tens of thousands of community members around the world, and with organizations ranging from small nonprofits to Fortune 100 companies.

In part I, I guide you in evaluating your social health with a three-step method, help you discover your unique social health style, and dive deeper into what social health is, why it matters, and what contributes to and detracts from it. In part II, you will glean practical steps you can take to bolster your social health; the resilient mindset that will help you navigate loneliness, rejection, and conflict; and inspiring examples of people from diverse backgrounds who are thriving thanks to connection. In part III, we travel to different countries and reexamine the world around us through the lens of social health—from our neighborhoods and workplaces to the technology, healthcare, and governments that structure our lives.

Taken together, this book is an invitation to see health as not only physical and mental but also social—and a call to action to prioritize relationships and community in your day-to-day life. It is also a manifesto for a movement centered on the practice of social health. This concept should not be confined to academic papers for researchers to discover and debate; it should be embodied and experienced by you and me and woven into the fabric of our society—helping us all live longer, healthier, and happier lives.

Whether you had never heard the term *social health* before picking up this book, or you want to level up your understanding of the art and science of connection, I wrote this for you.

Part I

ASSESS

The Fundamentals of Social Health

Chapter 1

Redefine What It Means to Be Healthy

Just like our physical and mental health, our "social health" is critical to our well-being.

—Vivek Murthy

In ancient times, people attributed headaches to demons and offered sacrifices to the deities in an attempt to cure their illnesses.[1] One hundred years ago, people smoked cigarettes without realizing that smoking could give them lung cancer.[2]

People's understanding of health has evolved over the course of history thanks to scientific discoveries and public engagement. These advances in how we *think* about health have also improved what we *do* to be healthy. Today, with modern med-icine, improved living conditions, health-focused legislations, and transformed cultural norms, you have a better chance of enjoying a long, healthy life than did any of your ancestors. Since 1800, child mortality rates have decreased from over 40 percent to less than 5 percent,[3] and the global average life ex-pectancy has increased by more than forty years.[4]

But this book isn't about our history; it's about our future. Further improving the quality and extending the length of our lives is not only possible but imminent. We have now reached another critical turning point in the evolution of what it means to be healthy.

Let's start by grounding the future in the present. The nar-rative about health that is most prevalent today, particularly in Western countries, focuses on two aspects: physical health and mental health.

Physical health, at its most basic level, is about our bodies. Ideal physical health means the absence or maintenance of physical diseases and the presence of physical strength and wellness. We can take care of our bodies to improve our phys-ical health through actions like exercising regularly, eating nu-tritious foods, getting a good night's sleep, and not smoking.

We all know this (whether or not we practice it), because it's common knowledge at this time in history.

Mental health, on the other hand, is fundamentally about our minds. Ideal mental health means the absence or maintenance of mental illnesses and the presence of psychological strength, emotional well-being, and resilience. We can take care of our minds to improve our mental health through actions like going to therapy, meditating, journaling, and learning to regulate our thoughts and emotions.

Mental health is historically newer than physical health in

our collective understanding, but is now a mainstream concept. Whereas my parents' generation looked down on therapy, for instance, most Millennials I know not only go to therapy but also talk openly about it.

Both of these aspects of overall health are vital and interconnected. When you strengthen your body, your mind benefits as well—and vice versa.

The problem is that they are incomplete. By primarily thinking of health as physical and mental, we are missing out on one of the biggest opportunities to optimize our overall health, well-being, and longevity.

When Robert D. Russell, the scholar I noted in the introduction, published his paper in the early 1970s attempting to define social health for the first time, he was ahead of the curve. Back then, there was solid research showing the health benefits of connection—but nowhere near as much robust, nuanced evidence as there is today. Back then, even mental health had not found its footing in public discourse.

The world wasn't ready for the idea of social health.

Now, in contrast, we've had fifty more years of advances in scientific research and people's understanding. As I'll describe later in this chapter, with so much data showing that connection is imperative for health, we can't ignore it any longer. Moreover, the COVID-19 pandemic and what many deem a loneliness epidemic have drawn attention to the importance of our social lives. In 2023, the US surgeon general (who is quoted at the start of this chapter) issued an advisory titled "Our Epidemic of Loneliness and Isolation." Advisories are national warnings about significant, urgent public health issues like smoking and drunk driving, which often mark turning points in American culture. With similar alarm bells ringing in countries around the world, we are ready.

It's time to harness this momentum and usher our understanding of health into the next era.

WHAT IS SOCIAL HEALTH?

Evolving and modernizing Russell's original definition, social health is *the aspect of overall health and well-being that comes from connection.* Whereas physical health is about our bodies and mental health is about our minds, social health is about our relationships. These three components are interconnected; even if you have a strong body and mind, you can't be fully healthy without meaningful connection.

Picture a Greek temple with three front columns, where the temple represents overall health and the columns represent the physical, mental, and social aspects of health.

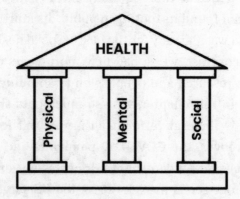

The columns support the temple by combining their strength. If you weaken or remove one column, you risk compromising the others and causing the whole structure to collapse. On the other hand, strengthening your social health can also help bolster your physical and mental health—and vice

versa. These different dimensions of health are mutually reinforcing.

To be clear, thinking of physical, mental, and social health
as distinct is a bit misleading because they are parts of a
whole that coalesce to make a healthy person. Nonetheless,
it can be helpful to consider them separately because the actions we take may differ for each—even though the benefits
extend to them all.

For instance, imagine a man named John who struggles
with alcoholism, which has taken a serious toll on his body
(physical health), triggered feelings of shame and despair
(mental health), and eroded his relationships with family and
friends (social health). John would benefit from a community
of people who empathize, don't cast judgment, and support his
journey of recovery. Connecting with such a community and
feeling less alone in his struggles would strengthen his social
health—and in turn help him recover and get back on track
with better physical and mental health, too. The strength of
one pillar reinforces the others. This is one of the main reasons
why Alcoholics Anonymous is so successful.[5]

Another example is exercise. When you work out, your body
feels energized, you get into better shape, and your physical
health improves. Your mental health improves, too, because
the endorphins released during exercise put you in a good
mood and you feel more positively about your physique. All of
this helps your social health as well, because you have more energy and confidence to socialize. The physical, mental, and social pillars support each other and together sustain the health
temple.

You might consider other dimensions of health and well-being
important, too. Some people might add columns to the sides and
back of the temple for spiritual health or environmental health,

for instance. Holistic health is multifaceted, and different cultures emphasize the importance of different components.

But for the most part, especially in modern Western culture, physical and mental health dominate the conversation and the rest is largely ignored.

That's a problem.

As we'll explore more in the coming pages, the social health column is so crucial to the structural integrity of the health temple overall that it deserves to be elevated in everyday conversations alongside physical and mental health.

The idea that health is not only physical and mental but also social might sound simple and straightforward—but its implications are profound. It means that if you nourish your body and mind but neglect your relationships, your overall health may be compromised. In contrast, prioritizing connection—in addition to habits that support your physical and mental health—can help you live longer, healthier, and happier.

WHAT IS SOCIAL HEALTH *NOT*?

Social health is different from the *social determinants of health*. This term, used mainly in the public health profession, refers to nonmedical factors that influence health outcomes, such as income, education, employment, and housing. These determinants are not social as in relational, but rather social as in societal, environmental, and contextual. While our relationships may be considered one kind of social determinant, thinking of them in that way understates the outsize impact they have.

Social health differs from social capital, too. *Social capital* describes the resources you have access to through your interpersonal networks. These resources could be emotional (such as feeling supported), but they could also be practical (such as advice or opportunities). The concept of social capital was popularized by Robert Putnam in his seminal book *Bowling Alone*, which sounded the alarm about the collapse of community in the US. Social capital contributes to social health.

Finally, social health is not simply about being social. Depending on your social health style, which you will identify in chapter 3, you might enjoy socializing casually at parties, for example—or you might find that draining. Either way, lasting social health requires deeper connection, mutual support, and a good relationship with yourself.

THE BUILDING BLOCKS OF SOCIAL HEALTH

In ancient Greece, builders constructed columns and temples using mud brick, timber, marble, and limestone. Similarly, your social health pillar is formed with various building blocks.

The structure is built up by your social life—who you interact with regularly, who you are close to, what relationships and communities influence you. As we'll explore throughout this book, it's not just your family, friends, and romantic partner who influence your health and well-being; it's also your coworkers, your neighbors, the stranger who held the door open for you, the barista you exchange pleasantries with.

All of these building blocks combine to make up the column. They are held together by your skills and tools—such as intention, emotional intelligence, vulnerability, reciprocity, conflict resolution, and self-insight. Signs of the column being strong include having the support you need and feeling cared for, understood, valued, and like you belong. Finally, the support the column provides to the overall temple includes myriad benefits throughout your life.

Let's discuss those now.

THE SCIENCE BEHIND SOCIAL HEALTH

There have been thousands of studies, with billions of participants, conducted by psychologists, neuroscientists, sociologists, and epidemiologists in countries around the world, that all point to social health as essential.

The problem is that they didn't have a coherent through line tying together this rich data.

One researcher studied friendships, another marriage, another family ties. One study looked at long-term relationships, another brief interactions with neighbors or strangers, and another connection with coworkers. One finding highlighted the benefits of being kind to others, while a different one focused on the benefits of feeling supported by someone else.

Now we can look at these and other research insights through a clearer, more holistic lens, realizing that they all add up to social health. In particular, three themes have emerged—three key outcomes of meaningful connection in all its forms: longevity, physical health, and well-being.

Before we explore these outcomes in more detail, note that the following is not meant to be an exhaustive overview of the research; that alone could fill (and has filled) entire books. Instead, the goal of this book is to reframe the conversation around social health and explore what we can actually *do* as humans going about our lives. What I've tried to do is share enough examples so that you have a solid understanding of the research and can use the scientific insights as a springboard.

One more technical note: I'll often describe the results of what scientists call *systematic reviews* and *meta-analyses*. A systematic review sorts through all relevant studies on a particular topic to summarize the main findings. A meta-analysis takes the data from numerous studies and analyzes it all together. In both cases, the goal is to draw an overall conclusion and distill decades of previous studies into key takeaways. By relying on these as much as possible, I've endeavored to highlight the highest-quality evidence.

With that, let's explore how social health can help you live longer, healthier, and happier.

LIVE LONGER

In 1979, two epidemiologists published a paper that would trigger a seismic shift in the scientific community's understanding of and interest in the link between relationships and life span.[6] Lisa Berkman, then at Yale University, and Leonard Syme at the University of California, Berkeley, followed nearly seven thousand adults for nine years. In that time period, men with fewer social and community ties were twice as likely to die—regardless of how physically healthy they were at the start of the study, their socioeconomic status, and whether they smoked, drank alcohol, were obese, exercised, or used preventive healthcare services. For isolated women, the risk of dying was closer to three times that of their connected counterparts.

This finding is astounding. It suggests that you are two to three times more likely to die in the next decade if your relationships are lacking, regardless of your other health habits.

In the decades since, many more studies have verified it. To examine them all together, a 2021 article in the journal *Frontiers in Psychology* summarized over one thousand one hundred studies with nearly 1.5 billion participants around the world (you read that right; billion with a *b*!).[7] The results were highly consistent. People with weak social health—measured by factors like the strength of family ties, the frequency of social contact, and marital status—were anywhere from 11 percent to 53 percent more likely to die from any cause. Similarly, a 2023 systematic review and meta-analysis in *Nature Human Behaviour* examined the health outcomes of over 2.2 million people aged eighteen years or older; those who were isolated or lonely had a significantly higher risk of all-cause mortality.[8]

In fact, researchers have calculated that when compared with other risk factors for death, lacking close relationships is comparable to regularly smoking cigarettes, excessively drinking alcohol, being physically inactive or obese, and getting exposed to air pollution.[9]

If you've watched *Live to 100: Secrets of the Blue Zones* on Netflix, this may not come as a surprise. Residents in communities around the world with the highest rates of centenarians—such as Ikaria in Greece, Nicoya in Costa Rica, and Okinawa in Japan—put family first and surround themselves with supportive social circles. To live a long time, we must cultivate meaningful relationships.

THE CAUSAL LINK BETWEEN SOCIAL HEALTH AND LONGEVITY

As a social scientist, I know it's not enough to say that people who are more connected also happen to live longer. We need to determine whether being more connected *causes* you to live longer.

That's what researchers in the UK set out to do. Since forcing one group of people to cut off their social ties, arranging for another group to have meaningful relationships, and then comparing how the two groups fare would be infeasible at best and unethical at worst, they had to examine the available evidence using guidelines that are commonly used to determine causality in health research, such as the link between smoking and lung cancer. This process includes evaluating the strength and consistency of the association and ruling out other possible explanations, for example. After a careful analysis, the researchers concluded that "strong social relationships *cause* better health and longer life."[10]

However, you don't just want to survive; you want to thrive. Social health helps you not only live longer but also be healthier and happier while alive.

LIVE HEALTHIER

As the Greek temple analogy shows, strong social health supports the physical health column. Connection in various forms is linked to a range of benefits for the body, including a stronger immune system, lower risk of disease, and greater overall health.

First, caring relationships can prevent you from getting sick in the first place. This is true for illnesses as minor as the common cold. For instance, one study showed that the more people felt supported and the more hugs they received over a two-week period, the fewer symptoms they developed when they were exposed to a cold virus.[11] (Quick tip: a hug a day keeps the doctor away!) Another study found that people with only one to three types of social ties were over four times more likely to develop a cold than people with six or more types of social ties.[12]

But this is also true for more serious diseases. Poor social relationships are linked to a 29 percent increased risk of developing cardiovascular disease and a 32 percent increased risk of having a stroke, which is comparable to other well-known risk factors like anxiety and job strain.[13] Overall, people who have a strong sense of belonging are 2.6 times more likely to report good or excellent health.[14]

In a now-famous study at Harvard University featured in the book *The Good Life: Lessons from the World's Longest Scientific Study of Happiness*, Robert Waldinger and his colleagues measured everything they could feasibly measure about a group of people for over eighty years to see what patterns would emerge. The main result came as a surprise to them: It wasn't the study participants' upbringings, educations, incomes, or lifestyles that predicted their health the most. It was their relationships.[15]

Meaningful connection also helps you recover *after* getting sick. Across different types of illness and disease, patients who feel more supported tend to experience fewer symptoms and even survive longer than patients who are more isolated.

For example, according to a systematic review of research on adults with type 2 diabetes, higher support from peers, spouses, family, friends, or healthcare professionals was linked to better clinical outcomes, including reduced blood glucose levels and lower mortality risk.[16] Programs that put this insight to use and include support as part of the treatment plan—such as having group doctor visits with fellow patients—have improved the health of diabetes patients more successfully than programs that don't include support.[17]

However, I don't want to provide false hope that love can cure cancer or other diseases. In one systematic review, investigators found that social support plays a significant role in the progression of breast cancer—but also noted that the severity of cancer was the best predictor of its progression, and factors like inadequate treatment, tumor size, and spread to other parts of the body were better predictors of survival than social support.[18]

Connection is not a substitute for medicine; it's a powerful complement to medicine. The experience and eventual outcome of a given illness are influenced by an individual's social ties: the stronger the ties, the better chance they have of staying healthy and recovering.

We all become patients at some point in our lives or know someone who faces a diagnosis. If you or your loved one is grappling with an illness or disease, think of social health as an essential component of the healing journey.

HOW PEOPLE GET UNDER YOUR SKIN—FOR BETTER OR FOR WORSE

A lack of love can quite literally break our hearts and harm our bodies. But how, exactly? How does the rapport you feel with another person shape the fate of your physical health?

One of the most popular answers to that question among researchers is that feeling connected to other people buffers against stress, which in turn mitigates stress responses in the body. These stress responses, such as heightened levels of cortisol, could otherwise weaken the immune system and lead to disease over time. For example, a 2018 meta-analysis of data from more than seventy-three thousand participants confirmed that those who were more connected had lower levels of inflammation, which is known to jeopardize the body.[19]

Let's dig into this more deeply. When we perceive a threat or experience a stressor—which could be anything from a saber-toothed tiger charging at us to a disagreement with a coworker—the body's defense system is activated. Prolonged activation aggravates the body, leading to cardiovascular and autonomic imbalances that are associated with morbidity and mortality. But our relationships can help us see threats as less threatening and more manageable, thereby quelling this chain of events.

For instance, in one study, participants consented to receive mild electric shocks while looking at photos of either their romantic partners or complete strangers.[20] When they looked at photos of their romantic partners, they reported feeling less fear, showed less activity in the brain regions associated with pain, and showed more activity in the brain regions associated with safety than when they looked at photos of strangers. (Quick tip: look at a picture of a loved one next time you get a shot or have blood drawn.)

Essentially, our relationships offer protection from the biological processes in our bodies that make us susceptible to getting sick.

They also influence the brain. Several studies, including one out of the Massachusetts Institute of Technology in 2020, have measured neural responses after people were isolated and discovered that the same brain regions were activated when people didn't eat.[21] In other words, loneliness is like hunger: a message from your body to your brain that it needs something it's not getting. Other research has shown that experiencing social rejection activates the pain regions in your brain.[22] We literally feel physical pain alongside the emotional pain of not belonging, of being cast out by peers.

Another explanation for all this is more practical. Other people can provide information or assistance that aids you in being healthy. For example, think of a compassionate doctor who takes time to explain and answer questions about your medications, or a family member who helps you monitor and keep on top of your medication regimen. The medication is what improves your health—but you need supportive relationships to take it correctly. Sure enough, medication adherence is almost twice as high in patients from cohesive families and worse in people who live alone or are unmarried, according to a 2004 meta-analysis.[23]

LIVE HAPPIER

The Greek temple analogy also shows that strong social health supports the mental health column.

Lexi is a nurse in Boston who I met through the Massachusetts Taskforce to End Loneliness and Build Community, a statewide coalition I collaborated with for three years. Lexi is used to taking care of patients at work. But in 2019, her skills were needed at home. When her dad was diagnosed with terminal pancreatic cancer, Lexi quit her job, moved across the country to be near him, and became his full-time caregiver.

As you might imagine, that was a challenging period in her life. There were many moments she cherished: spending quality time with her dad in his final months, taking pride in knowing how to advocate for him, giving him the best possible care. But there was also grief, anxiety, and loneliness. Lexi was twenty-seven years old at the time and felt as if she were the only person her age grappling with the responsibility of a dying family member.

In the darkest moments, she considered ending her own life.

For Lexi, the crucial element missing in her health was feeling understood and supported by people who knew firsthand what she was going through. Thankfully, she got referred to a program called ARCHANGELS that introduces caregivers to each other by phone. Being able to talk with other people in a similar situation provided instant solace and relief. She learned that one in four caregivers are Millennials, which helped her feel less alone.

"The moment I connected with them, I felt like I had a tribe behind me," Lexi told me. "Having support not only made me a better caregiver because I was taken care of; it also helped me be present with my father, appreciate the time we had together, and get a lot of meaning out of a really trying time."

While she drew strength from fellow caregivers, friends and family can also be helpful to lean on—but that requires vulnerability. "In hindsight, I wish I had allowed the people in my life to be there for me," Lexi continued. "I wish I had been more honest and had given them opportunities to support me."

In a 2018 systematic review, researchers synthesized previous studies on what helped caregivers cope, and they came to the same conclusion Lexi did: Social support enabled better psychological adjustment and less distress. Caregivers who socialized regularly, shared their experiences, and got help from friends, family members, and professional services were better off.[24]

Lexi's experience illustrates how connecting with others—and feeling understood and cared for by them—can help alleviate stress, build resilience, and stave off thoughts and intentions of suicide.

This is true for everyone, not just caregivers. One study in England found that the loneliest people in their nationally representative sample had up to seventeen times the odds of attempting suicide in the previous year than those who were less lonely.[25] Likewise, a 2015 systematic review reported that perceiving emotional support, receiving practical help, and having a large, diverse social network all buffer against depression.[26]

But couldn't it be that depressed people disconnect from their family and friends—rather than the opposite, that disconnection triggers depression? To find out, researchers at the University of Chicago followed a diverse group of people in their fifties and sixties over a five-year period. They discovered that loneliness predicted future changes in depressive symptoms, but not vice versa—which suggests that feeling lonely *causes* depression.[27] Another study showed a similar trend in children and adolescents: those with higher levels of social support demonstrated lower levels of depressive tendencies five years later.[28] Further building on this idea, researchers in New Zealand examined data on over twenty thousand adults and revealed that the extent to which people felt connected more strongly and more consistently predicted mental health than the other way around.[29]

All of this indicates that poor social health can cause poor mental health.

Interestingly, relationships reach further than our emotions, into the very functioning of our minds. According to a 2015 systematic review and meta-analysis, investigators found that infrequent social interaction significantly increased one's risk of developing dementia.[30] Among chronically isolated or lonely older adults, this amounts to a 49–60 percent higher risk—comparable to other well-established risk factors like depression, diabetes, hypertension, lack of education, physical inactivity, and smoking.[31]

In other words, having close relationships seems to be as important as exercising and not smoking when it comes to maintaining our cognitive abilities as we age.

A HAPPY LIFE IS A CONNECTED LIFE

Think about the last positive interaction you had with someone, such as dinner with your spouse or a phone call with a close friend. How did it make you feel?

Probably *happy*.

Similarly, reflect on a time in your life when you were embedded in the community around you and familiar with the people in it—perhaps while away at summer camp as a kid, living in a dorm while attending college, working at a certain job, or being active in a hobby or social group you belonged to. How would you describe that time in your life?

Probably happy, too.

Each year, the United Nations' Sustainable Development Solutions Network publishes a report on the state of happiness in 149 countries around the world. In 2021, amid the pandemic, the findings were unsurprisingly dismal—but also offered insight into which factors helped people experience joy despite the difficult circumstances.

One of the main factors? You guessed it: connection. Both the quantity and the quality of relationships were protective, as was living with a partner. Loneliness, a lack of social support, and living alone were associated with lower psychological well-being.[32]

Countless past studies echo these findings. In the *Oxford Handbook of Happiness*, researchers at the University of California, Los Angeles, noted that happiness is linked to the amount of time people spend socializing and how many friends they have.[33] But it's not just the numbers that matter. When people enjoy the time they spend socializing and feel satisfied with their friendships, they experience even greater happiness. This is true with romance, too. People are typically happy being married. But if they're *happily* married, they're even happier.

Importantly, the joy that comes from close, positive relationships can be enduring rather than fleeting. More connected people rate their overall life satisfaction as higher and benefit from a deeper sense of meaning and purpose. They tend to feel more optimistic about the future and be less prone to burnout.

As these findings show, a happy life is a connected life.

PLEASE DON'T DESPAIR

Perhaps you are now thinking, "I don't feel very connected—am I doomed to be miserable, get sick, and die early?" I want you to know the stakes are high so that you take social health seriously. But I have good news: there are proven steps you can take to expand your social circles (even if you're an introvert), deepen your relationships (even if you live far apart), and transform your social health overall.

Just as you can go from overweight to strong through regular exercise, from malnourished to healthy through nutritious diet, or from exhausted to rested through sleep habits, you can go from feeling isolated and lonely to connected and flourishing. You can also go from overly connected or stuck in negative relationship spirals to grounded in yourself and surrounded by positive support.

This book will show you how.

WHY THE LANGUAGE OF SOCIAL HEALTH IS POWERFUL

The unifying theme that integrates all the foregoing research is social health. The takeaway is this: We need to invest in our ties to friends, family, and community as if our lives depend on it— because they do. We need to elevate social health to be on par with physical and mental health—because it is.

We're not doing that, though. So what's holding us back?

WE UNDERVALUE THE IMPACT OF CONNECTION

Most people underestimate the importance of relationships for their health.

In 2018, researchers surveyed people in the US and UK about how they perceived various factors that influence life expectancy, such as smoking, alcohol consumption, exercise, obesity, and social support. They found that people perceived the relational factors as far less important for health than they actually are.[34] This was especially true among men, younger participants, and participants with a lower level of education. Similarly, another study showed that people in the US, UK, and Australia ranked physical activity and healthy weight as the biggest predictors of mortality risk, when their actual ranking was lower. In contrast, people ranked social integration and social support as low—when in fact they were the number one and number two biggest predictors of mortality risk in the researchers' analysis.[35] Perhaps unsurprisingly, then, in the US and UK, four in five people who often or always feel isolated, lonely, or left out, or who lack companionship do not recognize their disconnection as a major problem.[36]

While the impact of factors like smoking and exercise are well known, we clearly have a long way to go toward a broad understanding that connection is a vital determinant of overall health, well-being, and longevity.

This matters when thinking about the individual steps that you can take to be healthier. But it also matters when deciding what issues the government and healthcare system prioritize. When Gallup, a global analytics firm that advises employers and leaders, asked Americans what they considered the most urgent health problem in the US in 2021, nearly half said COVID-19.[37] Other common answers were healthcare access and affordability, while some people pointed to specific conditions like obesity, cancer, mental illness, and heart disease. To be sure, these are all important health problems.

But loneliness was not top of mind—despite the fact that it was deemed a public health epidemic by the US surgeon general, Vivek Murthy, in 2017. Despite 36 percent of all Americans, including 61 percent of young adults and 51 percent of mothers with small children, experiencing "serious loneliness" at the time of the Gallup survey.[38] Despite the health consequences of isolation among older adults costing the federal government close to $7 billion annually and lonely workers costing the US economy an estimated $406 billion in lost productivity.[39]

When I first read these findings, I wondered *why* people underestimate relationships so drastically. A simple Google search on "healthy habits" gave me an important clue. The top results were articles from reputable sources of health information like Harvard Medical School, the National Institutes of Health, the Cleveland Clinic, and WebMD containing many useful tips: Exercise regularly. Eat vegetables. Get a good night's sleep. Don't smoke. Drink water.

However, not one mentioned anything about relationships. People don't realize that connection is a health habit because it's missing from the prevailing narrative of what it means to be healthy. Even major, reputable sources of health information and experts in the health field tend to undervalue it or disregard it entirely.

At best, this is a missed opportunity. At worst, it is deadly.

When we take this all in, a few objectives become clear. One is that we need to help more people understand that human connection is necessary—not "nice to have"—for health. Another is that we need to translate that awareness into action, giving people the tools to be healthier through their relationships and setting up our society in such a way that connection and community are the norm.

That's what social health as an idea and approach can do.

MENTAL HEALTH IS NOT ENOUGH

The second reason that the language of social health is powerful is that it gives relationships the credit they deserve.

In the rare instances that connection *is* mentioned as a healthy habit in news outlets or expert advice, it is typically framed as benefiting emotional well-being—not physical health or longevity. The wide-reaching significance of relationships is overlooked and underappreciated because it has been buried in the conversation on mental health.

This is a huge problem.

People instinctively understand that quality relationships are good for mental health. Of course we feel happier and more resilient when we are supported by the people around us; that makes sense. But as we've just discussed, the advantages extend far beyond that to include susceptibility to disease and likelihood of dying. This fact gets lost if we keep discounting connection as just one of many factors for mental health.

By distinguishing and elevating social health, we can acknowledge how essential connection is while building on the mental model of health that we're already familiar with—extending it from physical and mental to social.

To be clear, I'm not arguing that mental health does not matter. On the contrary, I understand the importance of mental health more than many. I began my career studying psychology and working as a research coordinator in the Cognitive and Psychotic Disorders Lab at Queen's University in Canada. In that capacity, I got to know people whose lives had been disrupted by severe mental illnesses such as bipolar disorder, severe depression, and schizophrenia. Mental health is an essential pillar alongside physical and social health that we would all benefit from strengthening.

At the same time, the conversation falls short if we talk *only* about physical and mental health—and we will do people a disservice if we continue to hide relationships under the umbrella of mental health. Human connection is so important, so influential for our overall health and longevity, that it deserves to rise from the shadows and stand tall in the spotlight. It should be a protagonist, not a supporting character, on the stage of health.

One way to clearly see how social health is differentiated is to break down the three dimensions by their focus, their goals, and the behaviors that enhance them.

Dimension	Physical Health	Mental Health	Social Health
Focus	Your Body	Your Mind	Your Relationships
Examples of Goals	The presence of physical strength and the absence of disease	The presence of emotional well-being and the absence of distress	The presence of connection and the absence of loneliness
Examples of Behaviors	Exercise, Sleep	Therapy, Meditation	Connection, Volunteering

At the same time, it's worth reiterating how interconnected these dimensions are. For example, exercise can positively affect both physical and mental health. Therapy can positively affect both mental and social health (studies have shown that overcoming social anxiety and self-limiting beliefs with a therapist helps people feel less lonely). Socializing can positively affect physical, mental, and social health. Back to the Greek temple analogy: strengthening one column supports all three.

By reframing quality connection in its various forms as essential for social health and elevating it alongside physical and mental health, we can better appreciate just how *much* connection matters for overall health. Then the question becomes: How do we take action to optimize our relationships to live longer, healthier, and happier lives?

WE NEED A POSITIVE FRAMEWORK

That brings us to the third reason why the language of social health is powerful: it is positive and asset-focused. Let me explain.

In recent years, loneliness has been getting a lot of attention because of how widespread and detrimental it is. Every single major media outlet has published numerous articles about it. Coalitions dedicated to this issue have formed in the US, Canada, Australia, Germany, the Netherlands, and elsewhere. I would argue that a "loneliness economy" has emerged, with hundreds, if not thousands, of start-ups launched to solve the problem.

I became actively involved in this movement before it felt like a movement. I chose to focus my master's degree in public health at Harvard on solutions for loneliness. I have written articles, given talks, partnered on initiatives across sectors, and consulted for companies big and small, local and global, on the topic.

After all that, I have a confession: I'm *over* loneliness.

Don't get me wrong; it's an important issue—perhaps one of the most important of our time. But I've become disenchanted by the focus on fixing what's wrong. We need to focus more on fostering what's right. Solutions for loneliness are noble and valuable, but I want to see more approaches to cultivating social health.

These may seem like two sides of the same coin, but we can look at the field of positive psychology to see how the positive side can spark ideas that the negative side misses.

Martin Seligman is a renowned psychologist and former head of the American Psychological Association. He is perhaps most famous for pioneering the science of well-being and founding the Positive Psychology Center at the University of Pennsylvania, where I spent the summer of 2011 doing research in person and then continued collaborating with for several years from afar.

In the 1990s, Seligman noticed a perplexing trend in the US and other wealthy countries. Despite the majority of people having access to food, housing, employment, and other basic needs, many were anxious, depressed, or suicidal. This was even true among highly successful individuals who, at least from the outside looking in, seemed to have it all. Too often, people whose bank accounts contained millions were emotionally bankrupt. What was going on?

Trying to make sense of this data, Seligman realized that while psychologists knew a lot about mental illness, they knew very little about mental *wellness*. Missing from the research literature and clinical practice at that time was how to be happy and resilient, rather than just less miserable. So he set out to study, document, and share the habits and mindsets of people who flourished. The field of positive psychology was born.[40]

In the decades that followed, this topic exploded in popularity, with researchers complementing traditional psychology research—which Seligman characterized as more negative because of its focus on what goes wrong with people and how to fix it—with research on what goes right with people and how to foster more of that. Outside the ivory tower, positive psychology gained attention in popular media, adoption among psychology practitioners, and criticism.

The key insight I learned from studying positive psychology is this: the absence of illness is not the same as the presence of wellness. Addressing the negative is insufficient without also promoting the positive. Helping people survive is just the start; we also need to help people thrive.

Seligman and his colleagues reframed the narrative by shifting the field from focusing only on addressing mental deficits to also focusing on developing mental assets. In doing so, he blew the lid off the range of possible interventions. Suddenly, it wasn't just therapy and medication that could help people feel better but also finding purpose, adopting optimism, practicing mindfulness, cultivating resilience, and—yes—developing meaningful relationships.

This relatively simple reframing triggered new ideas, new research, new programs, and new tools that psychologists could add to their repertoires and the general public could use while going about their days—ones that might otherwise have been disregarded if considered at all. It was revolutionary.

That's what social health has the potential to do for relationships: generate new ideas, new research, new programs, and new tools to help people live more meaningfully connected, healthier lives. The language of social health is powerful because it points to three key mindsets.

Social health is inclusive and inviting. Not everyone is lonely, but everyone can benefit from cultivating connection and community. We all need to move our bodies, eat nutritious foods, and get restful sleep—not just people who are sick. In the same way, we all need to spend time with loved ones and feel cared for—not just people who are lonely.

Social health is positive and generative. It's an asset to invest in, a resource to cultivate, a source of not just surviving but also thriving. You don't want to go through your days barely scraping by, living but not enjoying life, alive but not healthy. You want to flourish. And you can't flourish without meaningful relationships.

Social health is proactive and preventive. Just as you shouldn't wait for a cancer diagnosis to take care of your physical health, nor neglect your mental health until you have an anxiety attack, you will benefit from strengthening your social health before loneliness even has a chance to take hold.

By redefining what it means to be healthy as taking care of not only our bodies and minds but also our relationships, and by recognizing that health is not only physical and mental but also social, we will move into the next phase of our collective understanding—and unleash new ways to maximize our potential to live long, healthy, happy lives.

Even for people who *do* appreciate the value of connection—even for those who recognize how essential it is for health—there has not been a clear framework for how to go about it. That changes now.

With this vision in mind, let's explore your personal social health.

Chapter 2

Demystify Your Relationships

We need joy as we need air. We need love as we need water. We need each other as we need the earth we share.

—Maya Angelou

How strong is your social health?

Before we walk through how to answer that question, reflect on a different one that you already know how to answer: How is your *physical* health? Maybe you can't recite your exact blood pressure or cholesterol level, but you know if you feel good in your body overall—if your weight is around where it should be, if you have energy throughout the day. You can sense when you're coming down with the flu or whether you've gotten stronger from working out.

It's noteworthy that there is not a single comprehensive metric that captures physical health—not one single score that sums it up neatly. Instead, doctors and other healthcare professionals look at many different factors to evaluate your body's well-being. They might measure your heart rate, temperature, and weight. They might ask you questions about your pain levels or symptoms. They might order tests like X-rays or urine samples to look at what's happening internally. Only by combining these inputs can they get a sense of your overall physical health.

You also know what steps you can take to be more physically healthy. It's common knowledge that eating nutritious foods, exercising regularly, and getting enough sleep are good for you, whereas smoking is bad for you, for example.

In the same way that you survey your body for signs of wellness or illness, you can survey your relationships. And in the same way that you take specific actions to strengthen your physical health, you can improve your social health.

HOW TO EVALUATE YOUR SOCIAL HEALTH

To integrate the third pillar of health into your life, you need to know where it stands now. So let's come back to the question: How strong is your social health?

I developed a three-step method for you to take stock and identify what you need to do to optimize. Just as your physical health evolves over time, your social health will change over the course of your life, so this method is about evaluating your current social health. The first step is to identify who fuels your social health. The second step is to reflect on the strength of each of those connections. And the third step is to decide what strategy would help you be most socially healthy. Embedded in the steps are guiding principles that will help you better understand what it means to be socially healthy.

At the end of the chapter, there is a worksheet for you to fill out that ties it all together. Let's begin!

STEP 1: IDENTIFY YOUR SOURCES

Exercise, nutrition, and sleep are examples of sources of physical health—what contributes to you being physically fit.

The *sources* of social health are what contribute to you feeling connected, and they fall into three main categories: relationships, communities, and other connections.

RELATIONSHIPS

The most important source of your social health is your one-on-one relationships with family, friends, romantic partners, coworkers, and neighbors. When I say *relationships*, I mean both platonic and romantic. Some of these relationships will be close and emotionally intimate, while others will be casual. All of them matter.

Reflect on the different relationships in your life.

Whose messages are pinned to the top?
Your inner circle of one to five relationships likely consists of immediate family members, close friends, and, if you have one, a romantic partner. These are the people who know you best

and support you, whom you trust, confide in, and care deeply about. These are often the people whose company you enjoy the most—and for good reason. As we've discussed, when these relationships are secure and positive, they not only engender joy but also are linked to long-term health outcomes like a stronger heart, enhanced cognitive ability, and a longer life span. Sharing experiences and spending time with these loved ones on a regular basis is nothing short of life-giving. If you have an iPhone, a fast way to identify these people in your life is to open your Messages app and see whose conversations you have pinned to the top.

Who is your emergency contact?

Among these, there is hopefully at least one person whom you can turn to in times of need. Recently, a friend of mine spent the day in the emergency room because of some unusual pains. While waiting anxiously for the doctor's verdict, he looked at his phone and asked himself, "Who can I call?" In that moment, he could think of two people whom he felt comfortable reaching out to for emotional support. Other relationships he cherished were with people he could laugh or discuss interests with—not call for comfort from the ER. He realized that each of his relationships offered different kinds of benefits. (Thankfully, his pains ended up not being a sign of something serious and the doctor cleared him to go home.)

Who feels like a spark for your soul?

Popularized in a 1997 book by the author John O'Donohue, *anam cara* is a Celtic concept of a "soul friend" or a platonic soulmate—someone with whom you have a deep,

mutual bond that transcends typical friendships. O'Donohue explained, "With the *anam cara* you could share your
innermost self, your mind, and your heart. This friendship
was an act of recognition and belonging." In my experience,
this kind of connection is rare and very special. Think about
whether you have someone like this in your life; if you do,
you're lucky!

Who is on your guest list?

Imagine you are planning your birthday party and need to
come up with the guest list. Aside from your inner circle, what
names do you write down? Your list may include extended family, casual friends, coworkers, and neighbors. These relationships also contribute to your social health, although often to
a lesser extent. These are the people in your outer circle who
you are not as close to—you might not tell them you love them,
for example—but who you either interact with regularly or feel
connected to in a meaningful way.

Who is *not* invited?

Not all connection is good connection. Disrespectful, negative, or even ambivalent relationships can detract from instead of contribute to your social health—actually causing
worse health overall—so deciding who to exclude as a source
may matter as much as who to include. As we'll discuss more
in chapter 4, you need to be selective because relationships
require time and energy. For example, if you're an extrovert
and say yes to every invitation to hang out, you might benefit
from focusing more on relationships with those who are most
important, like your partner or family. If you're a busy profes-

sional, it might not be a good use of your time to accept every request to "pick your brain" or network in your industry. On the extreme end, you may have to draw boundaries or let go of people who are abusive or toxic because they diminish your social health.

Do you have enough—or too many—sources?
If you find yourself alone more often than you want to be, or if you feel spread too thin, unable to give your loved ones the attention they deserve, you may need to recalibrate. Start monitoring this as you go about your days.

COMMUNITIES
Now let's examine the second key category of social health sources: groups.

A study of over twenty-five million Canadians found that a positive sense of belonging to one's local community was linked to better health outcomes, even after ruling out the effects of geography and socioeconomic status.[1] Another study collected data for over ten years from more than eleven thousand elderly individuals in Japan, revealing that perceptions of close community relationships and cohesion were associated with a reduced risk of mortality from cardiovascular disease, pulmonary disease, and all other causes.[2] Researchers have also discovered that the more groups an individual belongs to, the fewer depressive symptoms they have over time and the less likely they are to relapse if they were depressed initially.[3]

Taken together, this research shows that we should recognize the value of groups for our social health.

All for One and One for All **Principle**
Social health comes not only from relationships with individuals (all for one), but also from belonging to communities (one for all).

What groups are you part of?

Many kinds and sizes of communities could fulfill this need: the neighborhood or country you live in; the school or workplace where you spend your days; a hobby group you are involved in, like a sports team or book club; your religion or place of worship; or certain dimensions of your identity, such as your generation, sex or gender, race or ethnicity, or sexual orientation. Reflect on what fuels your personal sense of community.

Do you feel like you belong?

Communities are nourishing in a different way from one-on-one relationships. At their best, they provide a sense of belonging to something bigger than you, a safe space to bring out certain parts of yourself, and the sense of comfort that comes from feeling connected to other people who share a commonality, even if you don't know those people. Groups may not engender emotional intimacy as a trusted confidant can, but they can help you feel less alone, provide practical support, and open up opportunities for regular interaction and the development of closer friendships. For example, networks like Alcoholics Anonymous, as I mentioned before, or online patient support groups for people with rare diseases can be powerful sources of social health.

OTHER CONNECTIONS

The third and final category includes the other, less obvious ways that you might feel connected enough to reap social
health rewards. These include casual interactions with "weak
ties" that we often discount, like greeting the bus driver on your
commute, smiling at the security guard in your office building,
chatting with other parents at the playground, or exchanging
pleasantries with the cashier in the grocery store checkout line.
Another example is reminiscing about and feeling connected to
people who have died; those relationships can continue to feel
meaningful long after the loved one has passed away.

These sources also include nonhuman connection, such as
praying to and cultivating a relationship with God if you are
religious, playing with an affectionate pet, relating to or being
invested in the characters in books and movies, and spending
time in nature to feel connected to all living things. Although
we will focus mainly on relationships and communities in this
book, it's worth considering the value that these other sources
bring to your life, too.

STEP 2: REFLECT ON THE STRENGTH OF YOUR SOURCES

Now that you have a sense of who and what contributes to your
social health, how connected do you feel to each source? What is
the quality of your relationships and the communities you belong
to? These questions capture the *strength* of your sources—how
close you are to them and how satisfied you feel with that.

It's not enough to know a lot of people. We need to go deeper.
We need to be *mutually* and *meaningfully* connected with our
main sources of social health.

Is your connection mutual?

When you first think about social health, you may think about connection as a feeling: love, understanding, and support from other people. But connection is also an action: reaching out to others, helping them, letting them know you care.

For ongoing rapport, reciprocity is essential. Researchers have identified give-and-take as key to long-term relationship development and friendship maintenance—which makes sense.[4] No one likes a selfish person who talks nonstop about themselves, for instance, or only reaches out when it's convenient or beneficial for them. That's not a true friend. Of course, who is giving versus receiving more support in a given relationship may ebb and flow depending on what you are each going through, but the net exchange should be mutual.

It Takes Two to Tango Principle

Social health is best when bidirectional; we need to both give and receive in our relationships and communities to lead socially healthy lives.

I had to learn through trial and error to strike this balance. When I was younger, I was the staunch giver—the person my friends turned to when they were upset. I'm a good listener, and holding space for others without judgment feels gratifying to me. This role was a large part of my identity at that time.

The problem was that the roles rarely reversed; I was seldom the receiver—but not for the reason you might think. My friends were (and are) amazing and more than willing to reciprocate. It was I who was unwilling to receive. Reciprocity in relationships, I learned, requires vulnerability. I had to disclose the struggles I was going through in order for my friends to support me through them—similar to Lexi, the nurse in chapter 1. Looking back, I realize I missed out on opportunities to deepen multiple relationships because I was too reserved and held back from sharing more of my inner world with others.

Is your connection meaningful?

We know from positive psychology that taking medications may help relieve depression but won't guarantee happiness or fulfillment. In the same vein, you can surround yourself with people, but that won't necessarily make you feel more connected in the deep, fundamental way that we as humans crave.

To truly know each other and care about each other. To be seen, understood, and loved. To see, understand, and love others. This is the innate yearning at the core of social health.

The opposite is also true: you can feel connected while alone. Sometimes simply knowing that you are loved can make a world of difference. For instance, research shows that children who have just one caring adult looking out for them and supporting them as they grow up end up being more resilient as adults.[5]

Quality over Quantity Principle

In general, the quality of your sources is more important than the quantity of your sources.

In one study, researchers surveyed people of all ages about the size of their social networks—including family members, friends, coworkers, and neighbors—as well as their perception of those relationships. They found that being socially satisfied was a better predictor of well-being than having a large social network, leading them to conclude that "it is the perception of relationship quality rather than the perception of relationship quantity that is relevant to reporting better well-being."[6]

That's not to say that quantity doesn't matter at all. Other data suggests that there may be a minimum threshold of three close friends needed to flourish.[7] In general across cultures, people tend to gravitate toward one or two deep bonds, a handful of emotionally close relationships, and around fifteen friends. Note that those numbers may be higher or lower than what you gravitate toward, and that's perfectly fine; in the next chapter we'll explore what is the right amount of connection for you.

As well, what matters for your social health may evolve as you age. For instance, one study found that the quantity of social interactions at age twenty and the quality of social interactions at age thirty predicted social integration, friendship quality, loneliness, depression, and psychological well-being at age fifty.[8] When you are younger, interacting with a large number of people is important so that you can learn social skills, form your identity, and figure out what social health looks like for you. As you get older, you know yourself and your preferences better and also have less spare time for socializing, so it makes sense to prioritize fewer relationships and invest more deeply in them.

Are your sources as strong as you want them to be?
Taking into account the principles *It Takes Two to Tango* and *Quality over Quantity*, you may or may not feel that your relationships and communities are as fulfilling as you want them to be. Remember that you'll have a chance to reflect in more detail and write this down in the worksheet at the end of this chapter.

STEP 3: DECIDE ON YOUR STRATEGY

You won't get physically fit without deciding that you care about your physical health and then taking action to be more physically healthy. You won't get socially fit without a strategy, either.

The *strategy* refers to what you do for your social health, based on how satisfied you feel with the quantity and quality of your sources. There are four main strategies: Stretch, Rest, Tone, and Flex. The strategy you need now might differ in six months or a year as your social health ebbs and flows.

We will discuss specific, evidence-based ways to go about each strategy in part II, particularly in chapter 5, when we move from the fundamentals of social health to the practice of social health. For now, focus on identifying what strategy you need at this time in your life.

STRETCH IF THE QUANTITY IS LOW

If you don't have as many sources as you would like, your strategy is to Stretch: *make new friends, join or build a new community, and generally broaden the number of people and groups you can connect with.* Signs of needing to Stretch include moving somewhere new where you don't know anyone, outgrowing past relationships, or feeling isolated or lonely. To Stretch, you might go to an event in your town and introduce yourself to at least one person, or you might download one of the many friend-finding apps that have popped up in recent years and schedule a friend date with someone new.

For physical health, you stretch your muscles to improve flexibility and broaden your range of motion. For social health, Stretch your social muscles to improve sociability and broaden your sources of connection.

REST IF THE QUANTITY IS HIGH

If you have as many sources as you need or want, or more, your strategy is to *Rest: maintain or scale back the number of relationships or communities in your life.* Signs of needing to Rest include being content with how many people or groups you can reach out to and connect with, not having enough time or energy for all your relationships, feeling overwhelmed by social obligations, or entering a new phase of life in which the amount of connection that fulfills you is different. To Rest, you might keep focusing on the relationships and communities that are most important to you while letting go of the others, reduce how often you reach out to certain people, or decline invitations to dinners or parties.

For physical health, rest is essential in between exercises and workout days to avoid injuring yourself and allow your body to restore. For social health, Rest your social muscles to balance solitude with socializing and to show up fully for yourself and the people who matter most to you.

TONE IF THE QUALITY IS LOW

If you are dissatisfied with the strength of your sources, your strategy is to *Tone: deepen your connections with your existing relationships and communities.* Signs of needing to Tone include wanting to feel closer to your friends or family or feeling that your social ties are not as meaningful as you hope. To Tone, you might share a struggle you are facing with a friend and ask their advice, or you might write a thank-you card to a family member who means a lot to you.

For physical health, you tone your muscles to strengthen and shape your body. For social health, Tone your social muscles to enjoy stronger relationships and communities.

FLEX IF THE QUALITY IS HIGH

If you feel content with the strength of your sources, your strategy is to *Flex: sustain the bonds you have formed with others.* Signs of needing to Flex include feeling meaningfully connected to people and groups, having good habits regarding staying in touch and showing people you care, and generally feeling socially healthy. To Flex, keep doing what you're doing, because it seems to be working!

For physical health, you flex to show off the strong muscles you've built. For social health, Flex your social muscles to enjoy the benefits of mutual, meaningful connection in your life.

How do you like to connect?

There are many ways that researchers go about measuring how connected or disconnected people feel, like the Social Support Questionnaire or the UCLA Loneliness Scale, but they are all self-reported. That's because social health is subjective. Doctors can't determine whether or not we are socially healthy solely by running a brain scan or measuring a biomarker; they have to ask us about our perceptions and feelings.

Similarly, people's preferences for social health are subjective and unique, varying from person to person—so how you go about your strategy might differ from someone else. To draw a parallel, you may have tried different kinds of physical exercise over the years and realized that you are more of a yogi than a marathon runner, or vice versa. Some people like rock climbing, others biking, others lifting weights at the gym. So it is with connection. When it comes to social health, reflect on what feels nourishing to you, decide on your values in relationships, and put that into practice—rather than aiming for a certain score.

To Each Their Own Principle
Social health looks different for each person based on individual preferences and habits.

Try this thought exercise: Recall the last interaction you had that left you feeling energized. Who was it with? What were you doing? Was it in person or online? This will give you signals about what is important to you. Maybe you prefer shared experiences like going for a hike or checking out an art exhibit—or frequent, brief communication through texts, phone calls, FaceTime chats, and emails. Personally, my favorite way to connect is through laid-back quality time with the people I love—hanging out on my sister's porch talking, running around with my nieces and nephews, meeting a friend for dinner, just the two of us. In between these hangouts, I don't need much.

In the coming week, pay attention to the ways you are connecting and what you like (or dislike) about them. Notice how it feels to talk on the phone with a friend, laugh with a coworker about something that happened at work, or have breakfast on the weekend with your family. Also pay attention to the little moments of connection—the friendly barista who asks how your day is going, the neighbor who waves from across the street.

Have your connection habits and rituals changed?
In 2022, my husband and I moved for his job to a new town in California where we didn't know anyone, a two-hour drive from our nearest family and a plane ride away from most of our friends. Whereas he goes into an office several days a week and socializes in person with coworkers, I work from home, communicating with my team members and collaborators over

Zoom and email. Although I felt emotionally connected to and supported by my sources far away, the physical isolation took a toll and I found myself yearning for more in-person interaction. So I wrote cards and put them in the mailboxes of everyone on our street to introduce myself. I enrolled in a local emergency preparedness class to meet more people in my community. I struck up a conversation and exchanged numbers with a woman in my workout class. When an acquaintance introduced me to someone and we hit it off, I scheduled frequent hangouts to keep growing the connection. Gradually and with intention, I started to make new friends nearby, get to know our neighbors, and build a sense of community locally.

As my experience shows, transitions like moving to a new city, entering or ending a romantic relationship, leaving one job and starting a new one, becoming a parent, and retiring may make you feel more or less connected than before.

What Goes Down Will Come Up Principle

Social health is malleable; it will ebb and flow based on your life circumstances and the steps you take.

Social health is malleable in the same way that physical and mental health are. One year, you might be in really good shape, with a workout routine you like, and you might generally be in a positive, happy headspace. Another year, you might let slip the healthy habits that keep you fit and hit a rough patch with challenges that leave you feeling sad or anxious.

As difficult as these periods can be, malleability is actually a good thing because it means you can change it. You can improve your social health through the strategies you employ and the day-to-day choices you make—whether or not you make time to call your parents, how present or distracted you are when eating dinner with your spouse and kids. You may not be able to control all your external circumstances, but you do have agency over your connection habits and rituals.

YOUR SOCIAL HEALTH WORKSHEET

To tie this all together, here's how to use the foregoing steps and principles to evaluate your current social health. First, I'll go over the instructions, and then there is a table for you to fill out. This is a personal reflection exercise that you don't have to show anyone else unless you want to. Plan to spend around ten to twenty minutes filling this out, so get a pencil and a cup of coffee or tea and settle in. For reference, there's an example of a filled-out worksheet in the next chapter.

1. **Identify Your Sources**
In the Source column of the table, list the top one to fifteen relationships and communities that influence your social health.
   - Include those who are important to you no matter how often you interact with them (e.g., a beloved friend who lives far away) and those who you interact with often no matter how important they are to you (e.g., a coworker whose desk is next to yours).
   - Don't worry if you don't fill up all the rows.

2. **Reflect on the Strength of Your Sources**
Rate your satisfaction with each source in the Strength column.
   - Ask yourself:

» Is this a positive source that contributes to, not detracts from, my social health?

» Am I as close as I want to be with this person or group?

» Do I interact with them as frequently as I would like?

» Does our bond feel mutual and meaningful?

- If yes, put down a check mark (✓). If no, put an x (✗). If mixed or neutral, put a wavy line (~). This is a simple way to visualize which sources are strong and which could be strengthened.

3. **Decide on Your Strategy**

Select the strategy or strategies you need to take, both with your social health overall and for a given relationship or community.

- Write your overall social health strategy on the line at the bottom:
  » Stretch if you weren't able to list as many sources as you want.
  » Rest if you listed as many sources as you want or more.
  » Tone if you have mostly x's or wavy lines.
  » Flex if you have mostly check marks.
- Write your strategy for a given person or group on the row next to them in the Strategy column:
  » If you put a check mark (✓) next to them, Flex by continuing to do what you're doing.
  » If you put a wavy line (~) or an x (✗) next to them, Tone to strengthen the source if it is positive or Rest if the source is negative and detracts from your social health.

Source	Strength	Strategy

My overall strategy at this time is to _____.

- Optional bonus step: For each source you want to Tone, try thinking of one way you can do so. (You can always come back to this as you get more ideas over the course of this book.)

A FEW REMINDERS:

- *All for One and One for All*: As you list your sources, don't forget to include the communities you belong to that feel significant to you, in addition to the relationships.
- *It Takes Two to Tango*: When you reflect on the strength of each source, remember that connection is best when bidirectional.
- *Quality over Quantity*: The number of sources you write down is less important than the strength of those sources. You could feel meaningfully connected with just a few—or lonely or overextended with many.
- *To Each Their Own*: You might prefer sticking to a small inner circle or socializing with a large network. And there's no right or wrong answer for how you enjoy connecting.
- *What Goes Down Will Come Up*: If you realize that you are not as socially healthy as you would like right now, rest assured that this book will equip you to change that.

After completing the worksheet, you're probably wondering: Now how do I go about my overall strategy? What steps can I take with a given person or group? That is the focus of part II.

But first, it's important to know what strong social health looks like so you know what you're aiming for, as well as the factors that help you thrive through connection or that hinder your efforts to do so. That is the focus of the next chapter.

SUMMARY

- A *source* is who or what contributes to your social health. Sources fall into three categories:
  » Relationships with family, friends, romantic partners, coworkers, or neighbors
  » Communities you belong to
  » Other connections
- The *strength* of a given source is how satisfied you feel with your connection to it.
- The *strategy* is your approach to optimizing your social health. There are four strategies:
  » **Stretch** to increase your number of sources
  » **Rest** to maintain or reduce your number of sources
  » **Tone** to deepen your connections
  » **Flex** to sustain your connections
- There are five guiding *principles* when evaluating your social health:
  » *All for One and One for All*: Social health comes not only from relationships with individuals but also from belonging to communities.
  » *It Takes Two to Tango*: Social health is best when bidirectional; we need to both give and receive in our relationships and communities to lead socially healthy lives.

» *Quality over Quantity*: In general, the quality of your sources is more important than the quantity of your sources.

» *To Each Their Own*: Social health looks different for each person based on individual preferences and habits.

» *What Goes Down Will Come Up*: Social health is malleable; it will ebb and flow based on your life circumstances and the steps you take.

Chapter 3

Reveal Your Social Health Style

*Human relationships are primary in all of living.
When the gusty winds blow and shake our lives, if
we know that people care about us, we may bend
with the wind ... but we won't break.*

—Fred Rogers

Let me tell you about my friend Taylor.

Taylor is the best friend. Not *my* best friend (I should be so lucky!) but the best at *being a friend* of anyone I know. She means so much to so many people that she has been a maid of honor or bridesmaid in thirteen weddings—and planned many of those friends' bachelorette parties, bridal showers, and baby showers.

I met Taylor when she joined the team at one of my past jobs. We collaborated closely on a major national project and got to know each other well over several years. She was the kind of coworker who would put a bouquet of flowers on my desk for my birthday or suggest we grab drinks after a particularly stressful day. After both moving on to different jobs and different cities, we've stayed in touch partly because we bonded—and partly because she is really good (better than me!) at staying in touch with friends.

In chapter 1, we talked about how social health is an asset, a resource, a muscle to build up so that you have it ready when you need it most. Taylor knows this all too well. In 2020, her dad was diagnosed with stage 3 pancreatic cancer, a harsh disease that only 12 percent of patients survive past the five-year mark.[1] Friends and family rallied in support, showering Taylor, her parents, and her brother with love and raising over $200,000 to donate to pancreatic cancer research. Three years, one invasive surgery, and several rounds of chemotherapy later, he is still battling it.

In 2023, a year after their wedding, Taylor and her husband vacationed in Hawaii to celebrate their anniversary and pregnancy, overjoyed to be growing their new family. Two weeks later, they got the news that any expecting parent dreads: a fetal scan revealed that their baby was not going to make it.

Later, deep in mourning and healing, she texted me, "My social health is what's getting me through right now."

Taylor's sources checked in on her often, not shy about bringing up sensitive topics because their bonds were already deep. This enabled Taylor to keep talking about her challenges and working through her emotions with people she trusted, rather than hiding or suppressing them. Her sources also found unique ways to offer support, such as creating a personalized playlist for her to listen to, making a donation in her lost child's honor, and sending thoughtful gifts.

A support system of caring friends and loving family members was Taylor's foundation of resilience through the ongoing stress of her dad's illness and the emotional and physical trauma of losing her pregnancy. Her relationships helped her body and mind recover—the social health pillar bearing the weight of the health temple and helping repair the damaged physical and mental health pillars.

We can all learn from how Taylor approaches social health.

WHAT DOES STRONG SOCIAL HEALTH LOOK LIKE?

In her mid-thirties, Taylor lives in Colorado near her family, but many of her friends live elsewhere. The worksheet that follows walks through Taylor's current social health and how she stays connected to each source. Note that for the purpose of giving you more context into her approach, this includes more detail than you need to write in your own worksheet.

Taylor's overall strategy right now is to Flex. She is an example of what strong social health looks like—but it might be very different from what strong social health looks like to you.

For me as an introvert, the number of close friends Taylor maintains and the amount of time she spends socializing is shocking. If I were to talk on the phone with that many people every day, I would feel drained—which brings us to the first lesson from Taylor about what strong social health looks like.

Source	Strength	Strategy
My husband	✓	Flex: We spend time together every day.
My parents	✓	Flex: We talk on the phone every Sunday, and I see them in person a couple times a month.
My brother and his new wife	~	Tone: We chat by text or phone a few times a week, but I'd like to get closer with my sister-in-law. I plan to start calling her more one-on-one.
My grandparents	~	Tone: We stay in touch by email, and I send them cards in the mail, but I'd like to see them in person more often. I will plan more trips to visit them this year.
My two best friends from high school	✓	Flex: We text and talk on the phone every day, sharing the ins and outs of our personal lives. We live far apart, so we see each other two or three times a year. I also mail them cards and gifts.
My five best friends from college	✓	Flex: We text every day, sometimes one-on-one and sometimes in group chats, and I talk to them on the phone once a week. We live far apart, too, so we see each other two or three times a year and exchange cards and gifts in between.
A group of fitness friends	✓	Flex: We text a few times a week, mostly about our workouts and fun memes.

Source	Strength	Strategy
A group of other college friends	✓	Flex: We talk by text or phone several times a week. We also live near each other, so I see them once or twice a month.
A group of former coworkers who became friends	✓	Flex: They live nearby, so I see them once or twice a month.
A group of casual college friends	✓	Flex: We talk by text or phone every few weeks. We live far apart but hang out as a group a few times a year.
My husband's sister	~	Tone: We text once in a while. This is a newer relationship that I want to keep cultivating, but she lives in another country. When my husband and I visit over the holidays, I'll spend one-on-one time with her.
My friends' kids	✓	Flex: We FaceTime a few times a month, and I send them cards and gifts in the mail.
My coworkers at my new job	✗	Tone or Rest: I'd like to get to know some of my coworkers better. Our workplace is hybrid, so some days I work from home and some days I go into the office. When I'm in the office, I can schedule more lunches and coffees. At the same time, I want to set more boundaries than I have at past jobs by fully unplugging in the evenings and on the weekends.
My neighbors	✗	Stretch: I don't know many of our neighbors. I'd like to drop off holiday cards this winter. I can also use our new puppy as an excuse to strike up conversations when we're out walking.

THE RIGHT AMOUNT AND TYPE OF CONNECTION

Being socially healthy means having the right *amount* and *type* of connection for you personally. Thinking back to the principle *To Each Their Own*, recall that everyone has different social health preferences and habits.

Currently, on a typical day, I spend time with my husband, text with my family in a group chat, and maybe talk one-on-one by FaceTime or phone with a close loved one. Unlike Taylor, the most I connect with a given friend or group is once per week. In fact, most of my closest friends live in other cities or countries, and we talk every few weeks or months. But when we do, it's at length for an hour or more. And when we see each other in person, it's concentrated quality time. We've known each other for many years, so there is a deep bond. I know that if I wanted or needed to, I could call them at any time and they would be there for me, and vice versa. I feel connected to them and supported by them, and I know they feel the same way about me. I also relish alone time and can go for long periods in solitude without feeling lonely.

My preferences and habits look different from Taylor's—and that's totally fine.

"I am the definition of an extrovert," Taylor told me, laughing, when my jaw dropped at her social calendar. But as we'll discuss in a moment, extroversion doesn't fully capture Taylor's style because it indicates only the quantity of her social interactions—not the quality. "My inner circle gives me energy, but not meeting new people. I'm lit up by the people I *already* have a connection with."

YOUR SOCIAL HEALTH STYLE

There is no one "right" way to have a healthy social life. In my research, I have found that most people fall within four types. In the diagram that follows, you'll see different styles of connection preferences and habits: the Butterfly, the Wallflower, the Firefly, and the Evergreen. The up–down axis is your preferred or typical amount of interaction on a spectrum from infrequent to frequent. The left–right axis is your preferred or typical type of connection on a spectrum from casual to deep.

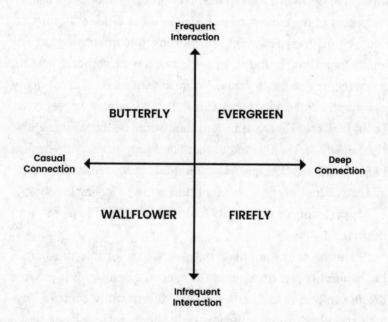

Butterfly

You thrive on frequent interaction and casual connection.

A Butterfly prefers frequent, casual connection, as do real butterflies fluttering from flower to flower to drink sweet nectar and pollinate the flowers in return. These people make wonderful party hosts and guests because they can mingle with anyone and will have fun making the rounds. This isn't to suggest that

Butterflies don't also appreciate deeper conversations and rapports, but they excel at and genuinely enjoy lighthearted interactions.

Wallflower

You thrive on infrequent interaction and casual connection.

In nature, wallflowers are plants that bloom in the springtime and then die back. Unassuming while growing against walls and in cracks, yet rich with medicinal properties, they were used by the ancient Romans and Greeks for healing. In social situations, these people are most comfortable with infrequent casual connection, staying out of the limelight—but they have the inner desire and ability to love and be loved, too.

Firefly

You thrive on infrequent interaction and deep connection.

I'm a Firefly, preferring infrequent but deep connection. In the wild, a firefly alternates between glowing brightly in synchrony with other fireflies and disappearing to camouflage with the night sky. In the same way, I need a balance of socializing and solitude. I love spending quality time one-on-one with loved ones or hosting gatherings for small groups of people. I also savor alone time.

Evergreen

You thrive on frequent interaction and deep connection.

Taylor is an Evergreen—a plant that is lush with green leaves all year round, not just seasonally. Being socially healthy to her means frequent deep connection, talking regularly with her closest friends and confidants. These interactions replenish her and her loved ones—just as the leaves on an evergreen plant store resources and nourish the soil below, which helps it and the nearby flora grow bigger.

ARE YOU A BUTTERFLY, WALLFLOWER, FIREFLY, OR EVERGREEN?

One style might immediately resonate with you or you may be a mix of more than one. Your style might evolve over time as well. A friend of mine was a Butterfly in his twenties, priding himself on being a loyal friend and loving son, maintaining numerous close relationships, and keeping in touch with everyone from high school and college. He socialized constantly, partied every weekend, organized brunches and dinners, and visited family often. Then, in his mid-thirties, he fell in love and got engaged—and his priorities shifted. He realized that in the next stage of his life, he wanted to be more of an Evergreen. His strategy changed from Flex to Rest: spending less time with casual acquaintances and focusing his energy on his closest friends and family. It meant that instead of planning a huge wedding with hundreds of guests as people expected, he and his fiancée opted for a more intimate gathering to celebrate their love.

One style is not better than another; they are simply different approaches. The Butterfly is not necessarily more socially healthy than the Wallflower just because they socialize more. The Wallflower may feel perfectly content with their amount and type of connection—although I might encourage them to Stretch or Tone and see how it feels.

AN INVITATION TO TRY A DIFFERENT STYLE

It's worth spending a bit more time on the difference between introverts (who could be Wallflowers or Fireflies) and extroverts (who could be Butterflies or Evergreens) because these personality traits influence the way we approach our social interactions and therefore affect our social health.

Psychologists define introversion and extroversion in various ways, but I like to think of them as reflecting a difference in energy: introverts recharge their batteries in solitude, whereas extroverts are energized by interacting with other people. At least one in every three people you know is an introvert; some researchers estimate that the prevalence is closer to one in two.

Contrary to the stereotype, introverts are not necessarily shy and reclusive; many, myself included, are outgoing and enjoy spending time with others—up to a point. Susan Cain, in her book *Quiet: The Power of Introverts in a World That Can't Stop Talking,* explained it this way: "Extroverts are the people who will add life to your dinner party" because they tend to be more gregarious, whereas introverts "may have strong social skills and enjoy parties and business meetings, but after a while wish they were home in their pajamas." Introverts still need and benefit from connection; that is a universal truth.

What does this personality trait mean for your social health? It will likely guide your number of sources: Butterflies and Evergreens typically cultivate larger social networks, whereas Wallflowers and Fireflies are content with fewer relationships and communities. It will also likely influence how natural or intimidating a given strategy feels to you; an extrovert may more easily Stretch, while an introvert is more predisposed to Rest. You can embrace your style if it makes you feel socially healthy.

That said, we can all benefit from pushing beyond our comfort zone, like lifting slightly heavier weights to get physically stronger. Consider a study published in the *Journal of Personality and Social Psychology* in 2020.[2] Participants wore unobtrusive audio recorders for one week and reported what interactions they had, as well as how happy and connected they felt, four times per day. The more often people interacted and the deeper their conversations, the higher their well-being—regardless of whether they were introverts or extroverts. The only variation the researchers found was that meaningful conversations helped introverts feel connected to a greater extent than extroverts—but both benefited overall.

So the message is this: be open to trying something different. If you are typically a Butterfly, Tone to deepen your existing connections or Rest by embracing alone time. If you are typically a Wallflower, Stretch to make more friends or Tone by opening up more. If you are typically a Firefly, Stretch by socializing more or Rest by making space for more casual interactions. And if you are typically an Evergreen, Rest to make sure you cultivate a relationship with yourself, too.

You might be surprised by how good it feels.

THE 5-3-1 GUIDELINE

If you're not sure what the right amount and type of connection are for you, you might need to experiment (we'll discuss adopting a mindset of experimentation in chapter 7). But insights from the research can serve as a starting point.

In particular, national survey data from Canada revealed what social habits correspond with the highest amount of well-being. The findings point to several useful recommendations.[3] First, connect with five different people each week.

Second, maintain at least three close relationships in general. And third, dedicate at least one hour each day to social interaction.[4]

Let's break these down a bit further. The five different people you connect with in a given week could include family members, friends, or coworkers, for example, and the way you connect with them could be spending time together in person, catching up over the phone, or some other way. Keep in mind the principle *To Each Their Own*: you have your own preferences for connection, and so do they. The three or more close relationships you keep are your innermost circle. Thinking back to chapter 2, recall that these are probably the first names that come to mind for the questions "Whose messages are pinned to the top?" and "Who is your emergency contact?" Ideally, the minimum of one hour per day you spend socializing is engaging rather than rote. Remember the principle *Quality over Quantity*: a few minutes of meaningful connection may be more rewarding than a few hours of being around people you don't particularly like or interacting superficially on social media.

These may not be exactly the right numbers for you, in the same way that not everyone needs to consume the same number of calories. If you're a Wallflower or Firefly, these numbers might seem high; if you're a Butterfly or Evergreen, they might seem low. But just as we're told to walk ten thousand steps, get eight hours of sleep, or drink eight glasses of water per day, guidelines can be helpful.

So use that rule of thumb: 5–3–1. Five different people per week. Three close relationships overall. One hour of quality connection each day.

At the time of this writing, researchers have partnered with the Public Health Agency of Canada, nonprofits, and an expert advisory group, in which I serve, to develop national connection guidelines, building on and expanding the available data. The goal is to elevate the importance of social health by educating policymakers, public health practitioners, and the general public.[5] Other leaders are working on similar guidelines, including the US government and the World Health Organization. Hopefully, more will follow. In the years to come, it's likely that you will learn about standardized social health recommendations where you live.

This is the same approach as the government of Canada's national food guide, which specifies how many portions of vegetables, fruits, grains, meats, and other foods one should eat each day. I remember learning about it when attending elementary school in Vancouver in the 1990s—and it works: more than 80 percent of Canadians know about the food guide and are aware that they should eat a balanced diet.[6]

If, within my lifetime, 80 percent of people become aware of social health guidelines and know how to cultivate mutual, meaningful connection, we will all be better off.

DIVERSE SOURCES

Another lesson we can learn from Taylor is the value of having diverse sources of social health. As we saw in her worksheet, she connects with her husband, family, friends from high school, friends from college, former coworkers, and various social groups. She and her best friends talk with each other every day, sharing everything about their lives. She also has casual acquaintances with whom she enjoys staying in touch in a more lighthearted way.

A series of studies led by researchers at Harvard Business School examined over fifty thousand people in eight countries and revealed that the more diverse a person's connections, the

greater the person's well-being.[7] Just as building a diverse financial portfolio is a prudent investment decision, they concluded
that building a diverse social portfolio is advantageous.

Moreover, the health benefits you get from each source may
vary. When researchers analyzed fifty publications with more
than one hundred thousand study participants, they found
that supportive family members contributed to a lower risk of
death, whereas supportive friends did not.[8] At the same time,
other studies have found that friendship has an outsize impact
on people's well-being later in life.[9]

This may be because humans have a range of social needs
that need to be met—including needs for advice and information, practical help, opportunities to care for others, reas-
surance that we are worthy, shared interests, and emotional
intimacy—which evolve over time.[10] Esther Perel, a popular
psychotherapist and expert on relationships and sexuality, has
pointed out that in modern Western culture, we often expect
our spouse or romantic partner to fulfill all of these needs—but
that's not realistic.[11]

For instance, being happily married is linked to better overall health,[12] lower mortality risk,[13] and higher life satisfaction.[14]
But a happy marriage is not enough (nor a requirement) for
a socially healthy life; it's just one source—you also benefit
from connecting with friends, family, coworkers, neighbors,
and even complete strangers. If you spend time *only* with your
spouse and let your friendships fall to the wayside, no matter
how wonderful that relationship is, you could end up feeling dependent and lonely. In that scenario, diversifying your sources
would enable you to indulge different sides of your personality,
explore other interests, and broaden your available sources of
support.

The same can be said for having one best friend. If you have one person who feels like your best friend, that's a wonderful gift. But you don't *need* a best friend to be socially healthy. In fact, it's risky to over-rely on any one relationship, whether romantic or platonic, familial or friendly. Instead, each one can be beneficial in different ways.

This holds true with coworkers, neighbors, and other acquaintances who you are not close to but see with some regularity. These weak ties often make up a community—and if you remember the principle *All for One and One for All*, you know that social health comes not only from individual relationships but also from broader groups that you belong to. You are linked to weak ties by virtue of being a member of the same community, whether it's your workplace, neighborhood, hobby, religion, or some other group. Even though you may not know each other well, you share that commonality.

It can also help to connect with people who you don't share anything in common with. Typically, we make friends by associating with people who are similar to us because that's an obvious way to relate to each other, familiarity is comfortable, and studies have shown that we typically like people who are like us. But breaking out of this habit can make life more interesting, not to mention affect long-term health.

Scientists in Japan compared people whose networks were similar to them with people whose networks were more diverse with respect to gender, age, race, ethnicity, socioeconomic status, religious affiliation, occupation, and other aspects of identity. Only the latter—having diverse networks—predicted health outcomes in their analysis.[15] This suggests that you can benefit from befriending people who are older or younger than you, have different colored skin from yours, or have a different belief system from yours, for example.

Look back at your social health worksheet. How diverse are

your sources, both in terms of the kinds of relationships and communities and in terms of their backgrounds? Could you Stretch or Tone with a greater variety of people or groups?

A SOLID FOUNDATION WITH YOURSELF

Continuing the theme of what strong social health looks like, healthy connection with other people requires a healthy foundation of connection with yourself. This entails knowing yourself, caring for yourself, honoring your needs, and bringing your authentic self into interactions with others.

One way to strengthen your relationship with yourself is through the practice of self-compassion, a concept popularized by Kristin Neff, a researcher and professor at the University of Texas at Austin. As she describes it, "Self-compassion is simply the process of turning compassion inward." Instead of being harsh and unforgiving to ourselves when we make mistakes, we can be kind and understanding. Instead of being critical and cold to ourselves when challenges come up, we can be supportive and encouraging. "Research indicates that self-compassion is one of the most powerful sources of coping and resilience we have available to us, radically improving our mental and physical wellbeing."[16] And, I would add, setting the stage for better *social* well-being.

This idea crystallized for me when I watched old family footage on a VHS tape. One video showed a little toddler in a diaper waddling around my parents' home on Easter, grinning from ear to ear while hunting for chocolate eggs. She was wide-eyed and innocent, so sweet and untainted by the world. I felt overwhelmed with love for this little child, wanting to hug her and protect her and make sure no harm came her way throughout her life—so much so that it brought tears to my eyes.

The little toddler was me.

Reflecting on this later, I realized the compassion I felt for the child version of myself was the same compassion I give to others—and the same compassion I should expect from others toward me. If we love and respect ourselves, we go into relationships more likely to love and respect others—and knowing that we deserve love and respect in return.

Think about your relationship with yourself. Do you carve out alone time? Do you treat yourself with the love, respect, and compassion you expect or want from others?

Of course, connecting with yourself is an ongoing process, not a one-time step to complete. Logan Ury is the director of relationship science for the dating app Hinge and author of the book *How to Not Die Alone*. Although she studies romantic relationships, many of her insights are relevant for platonic relationships, too. Logan told me there are two opposing beliefs she has come across in her work: one says you need to be a complete person before you find a partner, whereas the other says finding a partner will make you complete. She believes the truth lies somewhere in the middle: "The best-case scenario is that you're growing and developing your relationship with yourself while also growing and developing your relationships with others."

BARRIERS TO STRONG SOCIAL HEALTH

Strong social health means having the right amount and type of connection for your style, whether you are a Butterfly, Wallflower, Firefly, or Evergreen—and sometimes exploring beyond your usual preferences and habits to Stretch, Rest, Tone, or Flex. It means cultivating diverse sources and a solid foundation with yourself.

But what gets in the way? Let's consider a few examples of barriers that might impede your ability to enjoy mutual, meaningful connection.

YOUR OWN LIMITING BELIEFS

Through my work, I get to have conversations with people who range from being as socially healthy as Taylor to feeling despair and desperation over their lack of close relationships. I've noticed a common trend among those struggling: often, their own mindsets hold them back.

Imagine a woman named Jane who has been feeling lonely. Research has shown that lonely people tend to be hypervigilant in social interactions and more prone to focusing on the negative than the positive.[17] Thinking this way influences how Jane behaves in subtle but detrimental ways, such as being more guarded, feeling self-conscious, doubting herself, and making assumptions about what other people think of her. In turn, she has a harder time connecting—which reinforces her initial gloomy outlook. Jane's limiting beliefs trigger a downward spiral for her social health.

For this reason, one of the most effective interventions for loneliness in the academic literature is addressing maladaptive social cognition, which means challenging beliefs that are either not accurate or not helpful. In Jane's case, a therapist could help teach her to identify the automatic thoughts that come to mind in social situations and view them as hypotheses rather than facts, liberating her to try acting differently.

But sometimes a limiting belief can be as simple as not realizing that you can connect more deeply with people—or not thinking to try.

In 2018, I hosted a community event that brought together

fifteen Millennials and fifteen "Perennials" (what we called attendees who were on the older end of the age spectrum) for an afternoon of deeper connection. I was fortunate to collaborate with Ivan Cash, an award-winning interactive artist, and Scott Shigeoka, then a design lead at IDEO and now author of *Seek: How Curiosity Can Transform Your Life and Change the World*, who facilitated the gathering.

We matched attendees, all of whom were strangers, into intergenerational pairs. Then we guided them through a series of conversation prompts, such as "Share your life story in four minutes," "Describe a challenge you are currently facing," and "What is one thing you are especially proud of?"

The outcome was beautiful. I watched as people who had never met before opened up about personal experiences, bonded over surprising commonalities (one pair discovered they grew up within a few miles of each other in another state), laughed, and even cried.

At the end, we put our chairs in a circle to reflect as a group. One younger participant commented, "I'm surprised by how little space there is in my life to have conversations that are so human with anyone. If this was the norm, we would feel so much more connected."[18] It occurred to him that there in fact *was* space for deeper conversations—he just had to go for it. "I'm wondering why I don't even ask these questions with my existing friends."

Consider what beliefs or blind spots may be holding you back from being as socially healthy as you can be.

THE DEADLY *D*'S: DISCRIMINATION AND DYSFUNCTION

In a past newsletter to my community of fellow social health enthusiasts (you can join us at www.kasleykillam.com/newsletter),

I described going to a baseball game at Dodger Stadium as a Padres fan. Decked out in brown and gold gear, I was a visible outsider in the crowd of blue. I was surprised by how self-conscious it made me feel—and at the same time by the sense of kinship I felt with complete strangers who were also Padres fans. "This is a classic in-group vs. out-group scenario," I wrote, using the social psychology terms for categorizing people who are members of your community and those who are not. "It made me reflect on how feeling like we do or don't belong can affect our social health."

Being booed at by Dodgers fans was something I could easily shake off, but one community member, Victor, responded to my newsletter with a story that is much more profound.

Victor recalled being a Black pharmaceutical manager in the late 1990s. "I always tried to make my all-white team comfortable talking to me about race," he told me, "so I loved it when they asked me why, at every national meeting, all the Black people got together at the same tables. I didn't realize it had a name until reading your newsletter (i.e., in-group vs. out-group), but I was really pleased with the opportunity to ask them back: 'What would you do if you walked into a room with thousands of people and 98 percent were Black? Who would you gravitate toward?'"

Victor continued, "After we had a good discussion, I closed with, 'So the next time you see someone who isn't integrating with the larger organization, go out of your way to make them feel welcome instead of assuming they are being standoffish. Now you know they are likely trying to find comfort with people who at least look like them, just like you would do if the situation were reversed!'"

Feeling like an outsider, whether because of the sports team you root for, the color of your skin, or another aspect of your identity, can be a barrier to social health. This is especially true when there are real or perceived threats of discrimination, such as racism, sexism, ageism, or homophobia.

For example, researchers have documented how racism undermines relationships.[19] At the cultural level, racism may create "us" versus "them" dynamics that inhibit community building, social cohesion, and unity. At the interpersonal level, racism can erode interracial peer relations, blocking the ability to form, maintain, and benefit from those connections. And at the individual level, studies have shown time and time again that discrimination is detrimental to targeted individuals' health.[20] This risk factor feels especially relevant at a time of racial reckoning in the US. In 2022, 70 percent of American adults said they worried about race relations "a great deal" or "a fair amount,"[21] while two-thirds were dissatisfied with the state of race relations.[22]

More broadly, dysfunctional relational dynamics of all kinds threaten people's social health. Imagine growing up in a home with parents who did not express love, being bullied by peers at school, experiencing physical or emotional abuse from your partner, or speaking with a coworker whose communication habits include gaslighting or defensiveness. You can likely think of at least one example of someone in your life who has had a toxic effect on you, making you feel disrespected in small or big ways.

Any relationship will experience conflict from time to time; that's to be expected. With family members and romantic partners, for instance, you inevitably encounter disagreements, frustrations, and hurt feelings. While difficult, these challenges help you to get to know each other better and, if resolved respectfully, can actually deepen your connection. The same is true with coworkers. If you spend years working with someone, you're likely to clash at some point. Expect and even try embracing it as an opportunity to learn, empathize, and potentially augment your ability to get along and work well together.

But when the negativity crosses a line, those people can detract from your social health—not to mention your physical and mental health. Strong social health includes setting and enforcing boundaries for yourself.

When relationships are unequivocally negative, estrangement can be the outcome. In his book *Fault Lines*, the sociologist and Cornell University professor Karl Pillemer reveals that more than sixty-five million Americans endure ruptures among family members in which two or more people stop speaking to each other entirely. As his research has shown, these ruptures can take a devastating toll not only on the people who are stuck at an impasse but also for their loved ones and future generations.

At the same time, I know from personal experience that there can be very good reasons for estrangement, such as abuse, toxicity, and irreconcilable differences. Unfortunately, sometimes the socially healthy thing to do is to let go of someone and move on. As we touched on in chapter 2, deciding who is *not* a source may be as important as deciding who *is*.

Ambivalent relationships—where you both like and dislike the other person—are an interesting case. I'll bet you can think of a relative, for example, whom you have conflicted feelings about. The research suggests that to be socially healthy, it may be best to minimize contact with them. In a series of studies conducted in both laboratory and real-world settings, researchers showed that interacting with ambivalent friends, family, and romantic partners triggered higher blood pressure, more inflammation, and faster cellular aging than interacting with supportive ties.[23] Sometimes you can't avoid interacting with these people—for example, if they're a colleague at work or a teacher at your kid's school—so the task becomes to manage it as best as possible and counteract how it makes you feel with positive connection.

Remember:

- *Quality over Quantity*: Not all connection is good connection. Give yourself permission to let go of relationships or communities that are more negative than positive sources of social health in your life.
- *What Goes Down Will Come Up*: If you are going through a period of difficulty with other people, know that social health ebbs and flows; lean on other sources for support and know that yours will flow again.

These are big topics—bigger than I can cover here. Part of the purpose of this book is to spark many more conversations about social health and the nuances of how to cultivate it—recasting issues like discrimination and dysfunction through this lens. Reflect on whether these barriers may be relevant to you.

THE PARADOX OF BEING PLUGGED IN

When my mom moved to Denmark for a year in the 1960s after graduating from high school, long-distance phone calls were far too expensive, so she spoke to her parents only twice: on her birthday and on Christmas. Snail mail letters were her best option to keep in touch with friends back home. In contrast, when she and I moved to France together for a year in the 2000s while I was in high school, long-distance phone calls were more affordable and everyone had email, so regular communication was much easier.

Twenty years later, social media, email, and countless other free, instantaneous communication channels have become so pervasive that the problem is less how to stay connected and more how to *disconnect*. Adults in the US spend an average of more than three hours per day on their smartphones,[24] and around seven in ten people use social media,[25] too often scrolling mindlessly instead of connecting meaningfully. According to data by the Pew Research Center, 95 percent of American teens use a smartphone and nearly half are on the internet "almost constantly."[26] The majority spend time with their friends online on a daily or nearly daily basis.

All this time plugged in to devices has mixed effects on our social health. On one hand, 81 percent of those teens say it helps them feel connected to their friends.[27] On the other hand, when students at the University of Pennsylvania restricted their use of Facebook, Instagram, and Snapchat to a maximum of thirty minutes per day, they experienced a significant reduction in loneliness and depression three weeks later, compared with students who used social media freely.[28]

Problems arise when we assume that connecting on URLs will fulfill our deep yearning for connection IRL. In 2021, researchers published a systematic review of studies on social media use, social anxiety, and loneliness.[29] They found that both socially anxious and lonely people often turn to social media to make up for a lack of connection and support in person—but they don't necessarily find it there, either, instead spending a lot of time passively consuming content rather than actively engaging with people.

Technology may seem like a salve for disconnection, but it is too often a toxin.

That said, if used well, technology can be a powerful tool for social health; we'll discuss how to use it in chapter 9. For now, start to be more mindful of when your technology use seems to help or hinder your social health. Ask yourself: Am I using the tools available to connect meaningfully? Or are they substituting for quality time in person with the people I care about?

THE WORLD SHUTTING DOWN

Without discounting how tragic and traumatic it was, from a research point of view, the COVID-19 pandemic presented an unusual opportunity to study human connection. If you are a Wallflower or Firefly, you may have fared better than if you are a Butterfly or Evergreen because solitude is more your norm. But no matter your style, the global pandemic likely threw a wrench into your usual social routines.

In many ways, people's relationships suffered. A survey of more than twenty thousand people from over one hundred countries revealed that the number who felt severely lonely jumped up by 15 percent in the early months of isolation and uncertainty.[30] The AARP Foundation and the United Health Foundation found that 74 percent of older adults in the US had difficulty connecting with friends during the pandemic and two-thirds had infrequent social contact.[31] Researchers at Harvard University reported that 43 percent of young adults felt lonelier as a result of the outbreak, concluding that the "global pandemic has deepened an epidemic of loneliness in America."[32]

But other data that tracked people over time found more optimistic results. In 2021, researchers examined the results of twenty-five longitudinal and experimental studies involving over seventy-two thousand participants. They found no significant differences in people's levels of loneliness or social support caused by the lockdowns.[33] Then, in 2022, researchers conducted a systematic review with meta-analysis, looking at data on over two hundred fifteen thousand participants around the world. They found a small increase in loneliness—but nothing as sensational as the media headlines would have had you believe at that time.[34] In fact, in a study that followed people aged eighteen to ninety-eight in the US starting before COVID-19 struck and ending when lockdowns were in full force, some people reported feeling *more* supported during the pandemic, likely because many people were being intentional and proactive about caring for one another (from a safe distance).[35]

These seemingly contradictory findings actually present a hopeful message. Yes, something as catastrophic as a rampant disease that forces us to stay apart does present a barrier to social health. Yet keep in mind the principle *What Goes Down Will Come Up*. Most people were able to overcome that barrier—and in some cases emerge on the other side more meaningfully connected than before.

YOUR SOCIAL HEALTH IN CONTEXT

As disruptive and devastating as it was for many of us who lived through it, the COVID-19 pandemic is one challenge in the long history of all that humanity has survived—from diseases and disasters to wars and genocides—and a relatively temporary experience compared with the enduring structures, cultural norms, and ideologies that make up a given society. This broader, more permanent backdrop influences your ability to be socially healthy in both good and bad ways, likely without your realizing it.

In Robert D. Russell's original paper that we discussed in the introduction, he offered a secondary definition of social health that had emerged in his research. In addition to a dimension of individuals' well-being, social health might be interpreted as a condition of society. He struggled to reconcile these two meanings.

Whereas he was puzzled, I see perfect harmony. Public health professionals use the *social-ecological model* to show how a given individual's health is influenced by many different factors, and it can help us make sense of Russell's definitions. Each sphere represents a level of society.

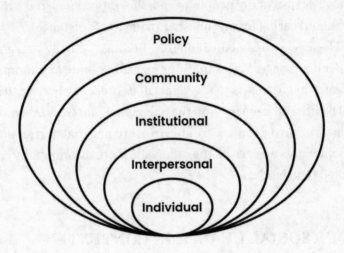

This model shows that you—and therefore your health—are embedded in the context around you, with individual, interpersonal, institutional, community, and policy factors at play. Each level presents opportunities to take action to address a given public health issue: from societal interventions, such as passing laws, to individual interventions, such as teaching skills.

For example, consider smoking. To reduce smoking, you could intervene at the individual level by educating people about the long-term health consequences. You could intervene at the institutional level by banning cigarettes in the workplace. Or you could intervene at the policy level by raising taxes on tobacco sales. Ideally, you would do all three and more—and we have, which is why smoking rates have decreased so dramatically, from over 40 percent of American adults in 1965 to less than 14 percent in 2018.[36]

If we apply this model to connection, your social health is determined by your own knowledge, attitudes, skills, and behaviors but also by the world around you. The interpersonal networks that you grew up with and interact with, the schools you enrolled in and workplaces where you spend your days, the community around you with its resources and norms, and the laws and culture of the society you live in—all of these influence social health. For that reason, the broader culture, institutions, and context within which we live cannot be ignored.

To bring this idea to life, let's consider three examples that could either pose barriers or highlight promising opportunities to improve social health throughout a population.

POLICIES FOR THE PEOPLE

Legislation can trigger downstream consequences that either inhibit or support your ability to connect. Consider parental leave, which is determined by the laws that govern the country and town where you live and implemented through the policies of the organization where you work. I currently live in the US, where parents typically get three months off to take care of their newborns.

In contrast, one of my close friends is German, and I was shocked to learn that she could take parental leave for up to three *years* after she gave birth to her daughter. This is the national law in Germany. After the first year, she opted to return to work part-time, but she maintained the flexibility to change her mind, knowing that a job would be waiting for her either way when she was ready. You can imagine how this generous policy enables her to focus on bonding with her baby, nurturing her and her daughter's health, and spending time with loved ones—all of which benefit her family's short- and long-term physical, mental, and social health.

No matter where you stand on the political spectrum, conservative or liberal, it's worth looking at a given issue or a given candidate through the lens of social health. What will the implications be for the connectedness of your neighborhood or country? Knowing that cultivating mutual, meaningful connection is a proactive, preventive approach to help individuals achieve better health, happiness, and longevity—which, in turn, helps society as a whole—what or whom should you vote for?

"ME" VERSUS "WE" DYNAMICS

Another example of your social health in context is whether the culture you live in is characterized as more individualistic or collectivistic. In general, people tend to prioritize independence and self-sufficiency in cultures that value the individual, as in the US and Australia, whereas people tend to prioritize interdependence and group harmony in cultures that value the collective, as in Brazil and India.[37]

Perhaps unsurprisingly, research has shown that individualism is linked to poor social health. For example, a study of over forty-six thousand people aged sixteen to ninety-nine in 237 countries, islands, and territories revealed that the more individualistic the culture, the lonelier its residents.[38] An emphasis on "me" over "we" can leave people feeling disconnected.

However, how this aspect of the culture affects your social health is not quite that straightforward. For example, some research suggests that people in individualistic countries may have an easier time forming new friendships and joining new communities, which is helpful if their strategy is to Stretch.[39] This could be because they are less attached to the social group they are born into. As well, the implications for health may vary. Surveying over forty thousand people in European countries, researchers found that loneliness took a greater toll on people's health if they lived in a more collectivistic country.[40] Presumably, feeling disconnected seems less acceptable and more shameful when you live in a place that puts such strong emphasis on family and community, resulting in worse outcomes.

THE RISE IN GOING SOLO

In recent decades, certain trends have shaped and continue to shape individual and collective social health. More people live by themselves than ever before; the number of single-person households has reached unprecedented highs in countries around the world.[41] Transience is common, with people relocating multiple times over the course of their lives. And, as mentioned in the introduction, membership in social clubs has declined. These trends do not *necessarily* cause people to feel more disconnected, but they are risk factors—and could be broader signals of devaluing family and community. That concerns me.

Taken together, these examples illustrate how social health can be a condition of society, influenced by policy, culture, trends, and other factors in the country you live in. It's important to consider these factors when we think about creating a more socially healthy world.

But to come full circle, social health is first and foremost an individual experience. Whether your strategy is to Stretch, Rest, Tone, or Flex, know that you have agency through the choices you make and the actions you take; the task is to figure out how, given the context around you. In part II, I will give you the tools to do exactly that. In part III, we will marry these two definitions together and explore what you can do beyond your relationships and communities, in the structures and environments where you live, work, and play.

Seeing your social health in context, considering potential barriers, knowing what strong social health entails, and understanding your own unique style—as we have explored in this chapter—will set you up for success. But first, you need to decide that social health is a priority for you.

Part II

ACT

The Practice of Social Health

Chapter 4

Make Social Health a Priority

How we spend our days is, of course, how we spend our lives.

—Annie Dillard

One of my favorite things about getting married was that I got a whole new set of family in addition to the one I already had. Nancy, for instance, is my husband's grandmother, and I am lucky to say that she has become like a grandmother to me, too.

Beyond that, Nancy is an inspiring model of overcoming barriers to social health and thriving through connection. In the span of her nearly nine decades of life, she has been resilient through ups and downs like we all face, but also through more extreme hardships. She attributes her well-being in her older years to social health.

Early experiences motivated Nancy to be intentional about relationships later in life. While she was growing up in a small town in Kansas in the 1930s and '40s, her parents modeled an engaged life, belonging to many social groups and regularly hosting dinners and card game nights at their home. Her dad worked long hours, but always put family first if Nancy or her sister needed help. In other ways, though, his love was difficult to decipher. At eight years of age, Nancy ran away from home in the middle of the night and trekked through the snow to the train station. When her dad found her several hours later, he did not hug her or express concern. Instead, they drove in silence until he pulled up at a boarding school for "problem girls" on the edge of town and told Nancy, "If you ever do that again, I will bring you here and leave you." Neither her mom nor sister said anything about the incident the next morning—or ever.

Later, as a wife and mom to five kids, Nancy moved to a new city every couple of years for her husband's job, which put stress on their marriage and made it challenging for her to form lasting friendships. Nancy made the best of the circumstances by fostering close relationships with her kids, creating a loving environment for them. But after most of her kids had grown up and had families of their own, Nancy's husband left her. In her late forties, she found herself having to open a bank account and earn income on her own for the first time.

While rebuilding her life and developing a career as an educator and school principal, Nancy made connection her guiding light. "I realized very quickly that I was going to have to do everything I could to keep us together as a family," Nancy told me. One of the ways she did this was by planning dedicated time for everyone to spend together, despite their busy lives.

The first summer after the divorce, she rented a home next to the Russian River for all her kids and grandkids to spend a week swimming, playing, and making memories. They returned every summer for fifteen years. "My kids remind me now that, if their dad hadn't left the equation, we would probably not be where we are as a family." Instead of divorce tearing them apart, Nancy made sure it brought them closer together.

In the years that followed, Nancy fell in love, remarried, and spent thirteen joyful years with a man who complemented her perfectly. Having navigated the reserved affection of her father, the frequent uprooting of her home, and the abandonment of her first husband, Nancy had found the warm, stable love she wanted. Then, unexpectedly and tragically, he passed away.

"There have been so many things that should have destroyed me," Nancy reflected one afternoon while we sat in her kitchen surrounded by Fourth of July decorations. Nancy's home is a cozy, creative wonderland. She lives there with her grandson Michael, and together they decorate the house for every holiday—and when I say *decorate*, I don't mean a few baubles, balloons, or banners. I mean every single inch of the house and yard is decked out with figurines, signs, garlands, artwork, and trinkets to celebrate the occasion, whether Valentine's Day, Easter, Christmas, autumn, someone's birthday, or another theme that tickles their fancy. Without exaggeration, they must have tens of thousands of decorations, brought out throughout the year to create magic for anyone who steps in the door.

The one kind of decoration that doesn't change is photos. Photos of Nancy's family line the hallway, sit on every shelf, and cover the walls. I knew I was considered family even before I married my husband when my photo made it onto the bulletin board in the kitchen.

The photos, like the summers on the Russian River, are an

indication of how Nancy centers her life around connection. Another is the calendar with everyone's birthdays and anniversaries hanging on the wall as a reminder for her to handwrite cards and mail gifts, which always arrive on time, if not early. Another is the bowl full of people's names, which she draws from each day to say a prayer and keep them in her thoughts. Yet another is the ringing of her phone, which is constant with texts and phone calls from all the family and friends whom she keeps close.

Nancy defies the stereotype of a lonely old person put out to pasture—and instead is a shining example of social health for people of any age. Let's look more closely at how she has done this.

CONNECTION AS A WAY OF LIFE

The first source of Nancy's social health, according to her, is God. Think back to the three categories of sources: relationships, communities, and other connections. Religious or spiritual connection falls under the third.

Not being religious myself, I asked Nancy to describe what her relationship with God feels like. "If you've ever had a best friend, someone that you could have over for a sleepover and whisper with until you fall asleep and tell your deepest secrets to and tell *everything*, every time you blundered, and they love you anyway—that's it. It is very, very personal. And I think it's made me intentional about loving other people."

That intentionality shows in her next most important source of social health: family. After one particularly thoughtful gift arrived in the mail from Nancy, I half-jokingly said to my husband, "I think we're her favorite!" He replied, "Yeah, except everyone thinks they are her favorite. She makes each family member feel so special and important to her, because they are."

Nowhere is this truer than with Michael, her grandson who lives with her. Both describe their close bond and daily companionship as a lifeline. They hug twice a day: once in the morning when they get up and once in the evening before they go to bed. "There is no way I could ever go back to living by myself," Nancy said.

Even while she was invested in her career, Nancy's family stayed her top priority. She cared deeply about education, growing the local school she ran from thirty children to two hundred and specializing in helping students who had learning disabilities and other special needs. "You can be passionate about something," she told me, "but you have to love more than your passion if you're going to be socially healthy when you're eighty-eight."

The next sources of Nancy's social health are the communities she belongs to and the friendships she has formed through them. She is actively involved with her local church, taking on the role of de facto leader as pastors have come and gone over the years. Sitting in her kitchen among the Fourth of July decorations, she described a conference she would be attending in a couple weeks that would convene church representatives from across the US to discuss modernizing their parishes and growing membership among younger generations.

Outside of church, Nancy has been hosting a group of women of different faiths at her house, and more recently on Zoom, twice per month for nearly thirty years. They call it Study, Prayer, Action: reading books, learning together, praying, keeping each other accountable in their everyday lives, and overall supporting one another. Then there's the COVID-19 recovery group of local women who meet on

Wednesday afternoons, the Bible study group with men and women on Tuesday mornings, the women who have stayed close after participating in a grief group for widows twenty years prior, and the friends from a Christian retreat years ago. This network has supported her through good times and bad, and vice versa.

Nancy is an active Firefly. As these examples show, she is extremely outgoing and involved, modeling to her children and grandchildren what her parents modeled to her. At the same time, she has cultivated a strong relationship with herself—regularly spending time alone painting, journaling, or reading. After a busy week of social engagements or the day after hosting a party, she likes to rest in the quiet of her home with Michael. "At eighty-eight, sometimes I think, why am I doing all this? But it's like second nature. I can't not do it."

Connection has become her way of life, reason for life, and driver of life.

PRO TIPS FROM NANCY

In studying Nancy, we can see the principles of social health at work. For instance:

- *All for One and One for All*: Nancy has many rich sources of community to draw from, in addition to the close individual bonds she has forged with family and friends.
- *It Takes Two to Tango*: Nancy has cultivated relationships that are truly bidirectional, such as with Michael. As an intergenerational household, they support each other, enriching both of their lives.
- *What Goes Down Will Come Up*: Nancy's social

health has ebbed and flowed over her lifetime.
Whether as a mom of five kids displaced every
couple of years or as a widow grieving the sudden
loss of her beloved husband, she overcame the
loneliness of these experiences by being deliberate
and consistent about nurturing the sources that are
most meaningful to her: God, her loved ones, and
the groups she belongs to.

As a result, Nancy is thriving. Despite being nearly ninety
years old, she lives in her own home, still drives a car, and is
proficient with technology. She has faced health challenges,
including a heart attack and diabetes, yet bounced back to re-
main physically active and mentally sharp. Her days are filled
with joy, love, meaning, purpose, and laughter. Nancy is one
of the most socially healthy people I know because she is intentional and proactive about it—and the benefits extend to
her physical and mental health, too: the pillars strengthen the
overall temple.

Nancy has made connection her top priority. And you can,
too, no matter your age. Here's the advice she shared with me
for living a socially healthy life.

RISK JOINING

Finding the right relationships and communities takes a little
courage. "Risk not being comfortable right away," she advised.
"Find someone who feels the same way you do about something. Find a group that supports the way you believe. Be true to
yourself, and risk joining. If it isn't comfortable and you don't
like it, keep trying until you do feel like you fit, until you have
people that speak the same language you speak."

FIND A COMMON THREAD

When Nancy's second husband passed away, she joined a grief group for widows like her. When she felt overwhelmed by isolation during the pandemic, she found a COVID-19 recovery group. "In every circumstance that I've been in, I've tried to find other people who have experienced the same thing," she explained. "That's the basis of every relationship: a common thread that connected us." Nancy turned to community in the wake of major crises, and it made all the difference in her life.

STAY INVOLVED

When her kids were young, Nancy ran the Cub Scouts club her son joined and became the director of the sleepaway camp her daughters went to. This level of participation has continued as she has gotten older, especially with her local church, where she constantly organizes events, fundraises, and even preaches on occasion. "When you retire or go through a major life change, do not hang everything up," she said, "Stay involved."

MAKE FRIENDS OF ALL AGES

"One of the things that happens in aging is you see people dying around you—your mate, your friends. If you just have old friends that you've had your whole life, you're going to lose them," she told me. "Regardless of your age, you need to be connected to people of all ages." What I love about this lesson is that it shows how malleable our social health can be—that it doesn't need to be stagnant or held to a certain standard based on a younger version of ourselves. We change. The people around us change. They even pass on. Give yourself permission to find new relationships and communities.

TOO BUSY TO BE KIND

In the Bible, Jesus recounts the story of a man who was robbed, beaten, and left to die on the side of the road. Both a priest and a Levite passed the man without stopping to help, but a Samaritan who saw him bound his wounds, brought him to an inn, and took care of him.

Inspired by this parable, researchers at Princeton University recruited forty theology students to participate in a now-famous study in the early 1970s.[1] Upon arrival, each student was told that they would be giving a short talk, either about seminary job prospects or about the Good Samaritan.

Next, the students were given directions to a different building, where they would record the talk. Some were told they needed to hurry because they were already late. Others were told to head right over. The remaining believed they had some time before they were expected. Regardless of the urgency, on the walk to the building all students passed a man who was slumped in a doorway coughing and groaning, clearly in distress. Unbeknownst to the students, the man rated them according to how compassionately they behaved—from not noticing him at all to asking whether he needed help or even insisting on taking him somewhere for comfort.

Overall, 40 percent of the students showed concern or helped in some way, whereas 60 percent either did not notice the man or noticed but did nothing. Surprisingly, the researchers found that being primed with the Good Samaritan parable did not affect the students' behavior. Instead, what mattered was time. Among those who helped, 10 percent had been hurrying, 45 percent were on time, and 63 percent were relaxed.

In other words, students who were less rushed were more likely to reach out.

This finding demonstrates one of the biggest impediments to making social health a priority: busyness. If you are preoccupied with your tasks, you have less mental bandwidth to pay attention to the people around you, let alone connect with them in a meaningful way. Connection requires time and energy, yet time and energy often feel scarce in modern life. According to the Pew Research Center, more than half of Americans say they are usually multitasking on two or more tasks.[2] Among parents of children under eighteen, nearly one-third always feel rushed.

If you often or always feel busy, it's worth pausing to ask yourself: To what end? What—or whom—are you so busy for?

CHOOSE TO DEDICATE TIME AND ENERGY TO PEOPLE

Since I first learned to hold a pen as a child, I have always loved writing cards. Over time, I've amassed a collection of beloved stationery, with paper and envelopes and stickers and pens in every color for every occasion—thank-yous, birthdays, holidays. I love the act of writing cards, and I love the result: someone I care about opens their mailbox and smiles, feeling connected to me.

Some years ago, I realized my box of stationery was sitting on my shelf collecting dust. At the time, I was very focused on building my career and was commuting two to three hours per day to and from the office where I worked. I had two to-do lists governing my life: my work one and my personal one. Every morning on my commute, I looked at both lists and chose the most pressing tasks, resigned to the fact that it wasn't possible to get everything done.

I stayed very much on top of my professional obligations. Guess what I never got around to? Writing cards. I was too busy to be kind—another way of saying I was prioritizing work over relationships.

But it's important to me to be the kind of person who writes cards, so I decided to reset by writing a card to every single one of my closest family and friends. My husband did the same. We wrote about memories we cherish and qualities we appreciate for each person. Reflecting on our relationships made us laugh at times and tear up at others.

Instead of mailing the cards, we put them on each person's plate when they gathered for our wedding celebration, so they read them in person with us when they sat down for dinner. Normally, weddings are about the bride and groom, but we wanted our wedding to be about connection with our community of loved ones. Several people came up to us right then with tears glimmering in their eyes to thank us. Many took the cards home as keepsakes. Of all the activities and surprises we planned for our wedding week, the cards seem to be what people remember the most—and they were what *we* enjoyed the most. The time and energy they took was 100 percent worthwhile.

Something Nancy told me that afternoon in her kitchen struck a chord and bears repeating: "You have to love more than your passion if you're going to be socially healthy when you're eighty-eight."

I have to admit, her words were a welcome reminder for me—even as the one writing this book. Like when my box of stationery collected dust on my shelf, I'm guilty at times of letting work take precedence over my physical, mental, and social health. On many occasions, I have moved far away from family to pursue job opportunities and stayed on top of professional responsibilities instead of staying in touch with friends, all because my career feels like my *calling*. Because I love my work, and work is a big part of my identity, it's all too easy to forget that in my eighties, more than anything else, I want to look back on a lifetime of love.

Are you too busy, or too career oriented, to be kind? Maybe cards aren't your thing. If so, think about what gestures of connection you do enjoy and recall the 5–3–1 guideline we discussed in chapter 3: Five different people per week. Three close relationships overall. One hour of quality connection each day. What do you need to do to hit those targets?

A LUXURY YOU CAN'T LIVE WITHOUT

When I have written articles and given talks about the importance of prioritizing social health, occasionally people voice concern that doing so is a luxury. One person wrote to me, "Sadly, as a community health worker (registered care aide), my work schedule is 100 percent anti-social, anti-family, making strengthening relationships one more benefit for only the rich." Because she was barely able to cover housing, food, and transportation costs, she elaborated, she had no disposable income or spare time left for socializing and hobbies.

This person raised an important point. Perhaps you can relate. If you are working around the clock to make ends meet, social health may be the last thing on your mind. You need to do your job, pay your bills, feed and clothe yourself and your family, and focus on basic survival needs. You're busy for a good reason.

Feeling too overwhelmed to invest time and energy, let alone money, in your friendships and other sources of social health is valid. Yet that may be precisely when it is needed most.

In part, that very sentiment motivated me to write this book. It's not always easy or feasible to prioritize social health in our day-to-day lives. Yet as the research tells us, connection is a necessity, not a luxury.

For that reason, I can't just write about what you as an individual can do to improve your social health. I must also argue that we as a society need to structure our workplaces, schools, governments, communities, and culture in such a way that social health can more easily become a priority. Thinking back to the social-ecological model we discussed in chapter 3, a person's social health is a by-product not only of that person's actions but also of the broader context around them. Our leaders have to set us and future generations up for success.

At the same time, connection does not need to be expensive or time-consuming for it to boost your social health. On the contrary, small steps that cost nothing can make a meaningful difference. For example, researchers at the University of British Columbia studied a scenario that you may participate in on a regular basis, if not every day: getting coffee.[3] Compared with people who rushed to buy coffee as efficiently as possible and get on their way, people who smiled, made eye contact, and briefly talked to the barista felt happier afterward. Turning an otherwise mundane transaction into an opportunity for joyful interaction is easy and free. We'll explore this theme in more detail in chapter 6.

With this in mind, I would invite that community health worker to think about how her interactions with coworkers and patients might be more connective so that the workplace becomes a contributor, rather than a barrier, to her social health (we'll also explore this theme in chapter 9). Outside of work, I would invite her to think about free, fast things she can do to maintain her relationships—such as a brief phone conversation with a friend while commuting to her job, a short stroll with a family member on her day off, or even a quick text message to someone saying, "Thinking of you." I would invite her to internalize the principle *Quality over Quantity*, focusing on the people or groups who mean the most to her and releasing herself of any pressure beyond that.

The task is not to complete an unrealistic overhaul of your life, particularly if you are already stretched thin. Instead, the goal is to make small adjustments that the data proves can yield big returns, in ways that feel realistic and joyful rather than burdensome. Here are some ways to go about making social health a priority.

EXERCISES FOR SOCIAL FITNESS

What comes naturally to Nancy isn't easy or automatic for many of us—myself included. Sometimes we need to be deliberate about connection until it becomes effortless.

Think about what feels feasible to you. If you are a Firefly, this might mean weaving rituals of connection into a busy schedule. If you are a Wallflower, it might mean small but mighty upticks in your social calendar, like joining a monthly book club at your local library. Experiment and play with it.

Just as with physical and mental health, we can experience meaningful improvements in our well-being when we make subtle lifestyle changes—think about taking three deep, mindful breaths each morning or substituting a cookie with fruit for dessert each evening. These rituals build on one another. And although they might start out feeling a bit like a chore, they become a way of life that we enjoy.

In my research, I have come across a variety of habits that meet people where they are as they start redefining health as not only physical and mental but also social.

NEXT TO YOUR TO-DO LIST, MAKE A TO-LOVE LIST

Good for any style, whether Butterfly, Wallflower, Firefly, or Evergreen

I love Nancy's ritual of writing the names of family and friends on slips of paper and keeping them in a bowl somewhere you will notice, such as on your nightstand or next to your coffee maker. She draws one each day to say a prayer for them and keep them in her thoughts. You could easily substitute saying a prayer with sending a quick text, giving them a call, or writing them a card.

Similarly, one of my friends keeps a sticky note inside his bathroom cabinet with the names of the people most important to him. When he brushes his teeth, he checks to see whether there's anyone he hasn't connected with recently, and he reaches out if so. Pick a place where you look regularly and call it your To-Love List.

ALONGSIDE CAREER GOALS, SET CONNECTION GOALS

Good for any style, whether Butterfly, Wallflower, Firefly, or Evergreen

You most likely have professional aspirations, such as getting a promotion, reaching a certain level of responsibility, or earning a desired salary. You may also have a plan for how to reach each of those goals over time. Why not bring that same forward thinking and strategic planning to your relationships and communities?

Envision one year from now, five years from now, and ten years from now. What social health milestones do you hope to reach? Maybe you want to commit to a romantic partner, make three new good friends, become closer with someone in your family, or be part of a local group that meets at least once a month. Whatever you choose, approach these in the same way that you would go about reaching your career goals. Make them a priority.

PUT YOUR RELATIONSHIPS ON AUTOPILOT
Especially if your style is Wallflower or Firefly
In aviation, pilots can set the plane on autopilot so that the flight path is controlled automatically rather than manually. They still need to pay attention and stay engaged, but flying the plane is easier this way because they don't have to use as much brain power on logistics.

Wherever possible, do this with your relationships. Turn on autopilot by putting connection on the calendar. Nancy's Study, Prayer, Action group meets at the same time on the first and third Wednesday of every month. This has gone on for almost thirty years. My mom sent out a standing invitation for Sunday evening dinners at her house.

What might you set up to make social health easier? Perhaps a quarterly phone call with a friend far away or a monthly meetup with a friend nearby. Maybe a weekly reminder to call a family member or check in on a neighbor.

MULTITASK AND MICRODOSE
Especially if your style is Butterfly or Evergreen
While riding the subway or driving to work, while taking a lunch break midday, while out walking your dog in the evening—those are opportunities to multitask and integrate connection into what you're already doing. Commutes are a great time to catch

up with a friend on the phone. When you need to run errands, think about inviting a family member to go with you.

It doesn't have to be a long interaction to fill up your cup. Taylor, who you met in the previous chapter, calls friends while folding laundry. "I think the pressure can build for some people, thinking, 'I haven't talked to that person in so long, it's going to be such a long conversation, I don't have time right now,'" she told me. "But you don't need to talk for an hour or more to feel connected. Just say, 'I only have 10 minutes but I wanted to say hi.' That can be enough."

It's important to not overdo it, though, so that you feel overwhelmed or distracted. This approach might not feel nourishing to everyone; as a Firefly, socializing requires my full attention, so I prefer to set aside dedicated time for it.

GO FOR CONNECTION FIRST

Especially if your style is Butterfly or Evergreen

Everyone has some amount of downtime or in-between time. Maybe for you it's first thing in the morning before your kids are awake, when instead of rushing to get ready, you could pause for just a few minutes to enjoy a cup of coffee or tea and connect with yourself. Maybe it's when a meeting ends fifteen minutes early, and instead of scrolling on social media or reading emails, you could think about someone you love and send them a text or give them a call to check in briefly.

Taylor juggles a full-time job with freelance consulting in the evenings and on weekends yet still connects with more people in a week than I do in a month. She told me, "I probably listen to fewer podcasts and consume less news than a lot of people. The news doesn't bring me joy. What brings me joy is learning about my friends' lives. So when I have downtime, the first thing I try is calling a friend. If they don't pick up, I try another. If they don't pick up, then maybe I'll put on a podcast. But I go for connection first."

Making social health a priority means deciding that it matters to you and being intentional about integrating it into your life in ways that feel feasible and fun. Even if this starts out feeling like a chore, it will become an enjoyable way of life—just like a muscle that gets stronger the more you work out.

Chapter 5

Strengthen Your Social Muscles

Friendship improves happiness and abates misery, by the doubling of our joy and the dividing of our grief.

—Marcus Tullius Cicero

In my senior year of college, I decided to conduct a personal experiment: I would do an act of kindness every day for 108 days.

I wanted to know: What will happen if I radically prioritize human connection in my life? What if I'm not allowed to fall asleep at night until I've connected with at least one friend, family member, or complete stranger in a meaningful way?

I chose 108 because of its auspicious meanings. To sports

fans, 108 is the number of stitches on official Major League baseballs. To literarians, 108 is the number of suitors who try to marry Penelope in Homer's *Odyssey*. To mathematicians, 108 is the product of $1^1 \times 2^2 \times 3^3$. To astronomers, 108 is the number of Suns that could fit between Earth and the Sun if you lined them up in a straight line—and, amazingly, also the number of Moons that could fit between Earth and the Moon.

But most of all, 108 is the number of prayer beads on a *mala* necklace. When I spent a month in a Buddhist monastery in Nepal two years prior, I learned to meditate with the *mala*—holding one bead at a time while reciting a mantra, repeating it 108 times in an effort to reach greater spiritual enlightenment.

In the experiment, acts of kindness would be my daily beads, my morning mantra, reminding me to set out each day with the intention of connecting.

Some days, the interactions were simple and lighthearted: smiling and striking up a conversation with a neighbor, complimenting a clerk at the grocery store, lifting a stroller up stairs for a pregnant mother. Other days, the exchanges felt profound. One morning, I left encouraging messages on sticky notes on the mirror in the women's restroom on campus. Incidentally, I returned to the same restroom that afternoon and discovered that someone had written a response: "No one looks at my face or talks to me. My life here sucks."

Her words jolted me. How many others were suffering, feeling unseen and uncared for? I wrote back: "No one should feel that way. Text me at [my number]. I'd love to hang out!" The girl never texted me—perhaps because she didn't return to the restroom and see my message, or perhaps because she felt ashamed. In the days that followed, I looked intently at every face I passed and wondered if they felt like she did.

I quickly realized how easy it had been to live a whole day

without doing anything for anyone else—not because I didn't care but because I was busy, absorbed in my own thoughts, goals, problems, and to-do list. I also realized how easy it was to change this. There were opportunities all around me to connect; I just had to act on them.

It felt as if my eyesight had been blurry without my knowing, and now I was wearing glasses that brought other people—and my relationship to them—into clear focus.

Over the course of the experiment, I connected with all sorts of people in all sorts of ways. I prioritized quality time and deep conversations with friends and family over assignments and studying. I got to know older women over tea at the nearby retirement residence and homeless men over meals at the nearby shelter. I schemed up ways to make strangers smile, such as leaving toys on the playground and spare coins in laundromats. I wrote letters expressing appreciation to various people, some of whom I knew well (like my mom) and some of whom I didn't know at all (like the janitor in my apartment building). I noticed a woman nervously waiting for an interview and gave her a high five and a pep talk. I saw someone collapse and comforted her until the ambulance came.

None of these acts of kindness were particularly special or heroic; what mattered was choosing to do them and making a habit of it. As an introverted Firefly, I would have been perfectly content sitting at home many days by myself with a book, not interacting with anyone. There were also days when I felt pressure to study for an exam or finish writing an essay due the next day, when serving others seemed as if it would be self-destructive. But I found that the effort was always worthwhile and didn't require a lot of time to be meaningful.

I also observed that spreading kindness came full circle. Late in February, my dad told me over the phone from Vancouver that he had been diagnosed with cancer. The next day was the fiftieth of 108, and in celebration I had ordered fifty helium balloons and recruited a few friends to help me hand them out to passersby in downtown Toronto.

Despite being upset and still in shock, I moved forward with the plan. Spending time with friends brought solace, as did being the source of so many smiles and laughs—watching everyone from little kids to office workers in suits disappear down the sidewalk with balloons in tow. That day, I needed the warmth of connection to offset my grief and anxiety. The point had been bringing joy to others, but doing so brought joy to me.

On the 100th day, a friend and I stood at the entrance to the college library with signs I had made that said, "Feeling stressed about exams? Have a free hug!" Despite having come up with the idea, I felt reluctant at first. After all, *I* was feeling stressed about exams, not to mention nervous about putting myself out there in such a visible way in front of peers. But several hours and hundreds of hugs later, I was on cloud nine. The energy from so many positive interactions vibrated in every cell of my body.

In fact, that energy infused my whole life. I conducted my 108-day experiment during my time as a research-driven psychology student at Queen's University in Canada, but it was intentionally less about formal data collection and more about observing how these choices and actions affected who I was as a person—my mood, my sense of self, my long-term goals and values, my bond with my community, and my well-being. Even without quantitative analysis, the results of my 108-day experiment were unmistakable.

I had hypothesized that my relationships would broaden and deepen, Stretch and Tone, and they did; I made new friends and got closer to my loved ones. I became more in tune with the people around me—listening more intently, empathizing more intensely—and also opened up more, inviting others to get closer to me. I felt deeply connected to other people, to my community, and to myself. As a result, my day-to-day life seemed elevated, with more meaning, purpose, and fulfillment. I felt alive.

At the same time, various secondary effects took me by surprise. My motivation to take care of other aspects of my well-being—like exercising and cooking healthy meals—increased, so my body had more energy and my mental focus sharpened. Despite having less time to focus on schoolwork, I was more productive and efficient and actually ended up achieving the highest grade point average of all my semesters at college. More interactions with people led to useful introductions and new ideas, opening doors to unexpected career opportunities. After 108 days of prioritizing connection, my life was better in just about every way you can imagine.

I didn't have the language to explain it then, but I know now that what I was doing was strengthening my social muscles and improving my social health—and thereby bolstering my overall health temple.

CONNECTION IS LIKE EXERCISE

One of the main messages of this book is that social health is as important as physical and mental health. Just as we take steps to be physically and mentally healthy, we should take steps to be socially healthy.

Think of connection as like exercise. In the past, I've

experimented with many kinds of exercise to figure out what I like best—going to the gym, running, swimming; when I was younger I did hip-hop, tae kwon do, softball, and fencing (don't cross with me with a sword). More recently, I've gotten into a routine I love of Pilates and CrossFit classes two or three times per week and walks on other days. Although it started out feeling like a chore, it has become a ritual that I look forward to, a natural part of my lifestyle that I don't think twice about anymore. Now, if a week goes by without a vigorous workout, I feel unwell physically and mentally.

In the same way, you can experiment with and be mindful of what kinds of connection you enjoy. Remember the principle *To Each Their Own*: social health looks different for each person based on individual preferences and habits.

With my 108-day experiment, I exercised my social muscles every day through acts of kindness. Connection was my daily workout. Admittedly, it was quite an extreme routine—that intensity is too much for me to sustain on an ongoing basis. But I learned that certain interactions felt more nourishing than others—and that being intentional about making connection part of my lifestyle is transformative.

HOW TO STRETCH, REST, TONE, OR FLEX

Refer back to the worksheet you filled out in chapter 2. Is your overall social health strategy to Stretch (increase your number of sources), Rest (maintain or reduce your number of sources), Tone (deepen your connections), Flex (sustain your connections), or a mix of these? Then try some of the following research-backed and Kasley-tested suggestions. These are meant not as a comprehensive guide, but as a foundation to build on.

HOBBIES: DO WHAT YOU LOVE WITH OTHERS
Especially if your strategy is to Stretch, Tone, or Flex

One of the best ways to strengthen your social muscles is to do what you love with others.

If you like hiking, find a local hiking group by searching on Meetup or Eventbrite, websites for finding groups with shared interests. If you like playing music, look up local bars that host open mic nights. Invite a friend to try pickleball with you or a neighbor to come over for arts and crafts. Whatever your hobby, there are others who love it, too—and that's a great way to bond.

This is how many of the people who received $1,000 microgrants from Social Health Labs, the nonprofit I lead, got started. The microgrants support local, grassroots efforts to improve social health in neighborhoods across the US.

For instance, Zaineb, a deaf Iraqi American woman in her thirties who lives in Chicago, loves coffee and introduced her friends to *qazwan,* a type of coffee brewed with the roasted seeds of pistachio trees. Several of her friends shared their own methods of brewing coffee from the countries they came from, which brought them closer together. Zaineb realized this could be a tool to bridge divides. She used a microgrant to convene Chicagoans of diverse backgrounds and hearing abilities to connect across their differences while brewing coffee.

Six-year-old Sebastian loved finding caterpillars in the garden and learning about their life cycle to transform into butterflies. He and his grandmother, Kathy, used a microgrant to set up habitats and stock them with monarch eggs and milkweed at senior living communities near where they lived in Wisconsin. Over the course of taking care of the caterpillars, watching them form cocoons and hatch, and setting the butterflies free, Sebastian and Kathy bonded with the older residents, staff, and other families—not to mention each other. The following summer, seven more families and a Girl Scout troop joined their efforts, leading to even more intergenerational connections.

As Sebastian and Kathy's story illustrates, consistency is important. You can't go do a set of sit-ups and push-ups one day, never exercise again, and expect to be strong. Your physical muscles need to be worked out regularly in order to stay fit. The same is true with social muscles—and with any given relationship or community. Research shows that time and intimacy have a linear correlation: the more time you spend with someone, the closer you become.[1] So make your hobby with others a weekly or monthly activity.

VOLUNTEERING: CONTRIBUTE TO YOUR COMMUNITY
Especially if your strategy is to Stretch

My mom grew up in a small town in Northern California nestled between the forest and the ocean. As a child, she ran around barefoot among the redwoods behind her house, the treetops disappearing in fog far above her head. As a teenager, she threw a surfboard in the back seat of her hand-me-down Austin-Healey Sprite and skipped school to ride the waves with her friends. Her love of nature is deeply ingrained.

Fast-forward to her sixties, when my mom started spending winters in Arizona. At first, she didn't know anyone nearby. Faced with building a brand-new network, and following her desire to explore the surrounding desert, she decided to get involved with the local nature conservancy. As a volunteer steward, she underwent training with a cohort of other retirees, becoming knowledgeable about the native flora and fauna and ultimately guiding groups on educational hikes around the preserve. Now instead of redwoods and waves, she navigates saguaro cacti and scorpions.

Through volunteering, my mom became part of a community of people who love being active outdoors as she does—and made new friends who have become close in the years since.

Those are exactly the reasons why volunteering can be a wonderful way to Stretch. In a study of nearly six thousand people across the US, recently widowed adults felt considerably lonelier than their married counterparts—until they started volunteering for two or more hours per week.[2] Other research has shown that the more you volunteer, the higher your well-being; this is especially true for older adults, who may have more flexible time to spend in this way.[3] But these benefits are true no matter your age.

If you feel lonely, volunteering can be an especially helpful approach. Loneliness is often a self-focused, internal experience. As discussed in chapter 3, it's easy to get stuck in a mental loop—thinking negative thoughts, feeling sad and alone, losing hope and motivation. For instance, studies have shown that lonely people tend to fall into traps like rumination, catastrophizing, suppression, and withdrawal.[4] Instead, refocusing your attention outward by volunteering and channeling your energy to help other people can help snap you out of that mindset. Plus, the immediate dopamine hit of interacting with other people positively reinforces the experience, making you want to do it again. Before you know it, you just might not feel lonely anymore.

If you want to meet new people and form new relationships, volunteer with a local cause you care about. You can find opportunities in cities and countries around the world through VolunteerMatch, an online database, or by reaching out to an organization whose work you admire to ask if it needs help.

CONVERSATION: ASK BETTER QUESTIONS
Especially if your strategy is to Stretch, Tone, or Flex

In 2018, researchers at Facebook (now Meta) and Carnegie Mellon University surveyed over four thousand six hundred people in the US, India, and Japan about what meaningful interactions, both online and offline, looked like to them.[5] A common theme was that interactions felt meaningful if they resulted in an emotional, informational, or tangible impact. For example, one participant described a conversation with their partner that made the two of them feel closer (emotional impact). Another cited giving advice to her daughter that she found useful (informational impact). Yet another talked about providing food and water to flood victims (tangible impact).

When people did *not* find a given interaction meaningful, they described it as "trivial," "not genuine," "small talk," or "only for timepass." Evidently, people in all three cultures were more fulfilled by going deeper, whether with loved ones or with strangers.

In 2015, I started a blog called *The Opposite of Small Talk* as a creative outlet and a way to experiment with human connection in my spare time. The premise was to strike up conversations with strangers in my community, testing how open they would be to bypassing casual chitchat and diving straight into personal topics. This resulted in a variety of beautiful interactions, but one person in particular I've never forgotten: Christos the cobbler.

Christos had nasty reviews on Yelp, which I had read because I needed a shoe fixed. I wouldn't have given it any more thought, except I passed his shoe repair shop most mornings on my way to work. I couldn't help but wonder: Was he as curmudgeonly as past customers claimed? Could there be more to his story?

One day, I decided to find out. The doorbell jingled as I

walked into his shop, past the walls lined with laces, sole inserts, and leather sprays, up to the counter. Christos came out from the back. He was short with a round face and a bald head, except for a tuft of white hair on either side, and he looked to be in his eighties. "What can I do for you?" he asked in a thick accent. I introduced myself and explained the blog.

"Would you be willing to share your life story?" I asked. To my surprise, a smile spread from tuft to tuft and he agreed.

Over the course of an hour and a baklava he brought out from the back to share with me, Christos told me about growing up in poverty in a tiny village in Greece, apprenticing with a cobbler starting at age eleven, falling in love for the first and only time, moving to America with barely a penny to his name, and eventually setting up his business. Years later his wife died, leaving him feeling depressed and suicidal. Christos described his kids and grandkids and shared his worries about how he'll fare once he's too old to run the shop.

All I had done was ask one question—whether he would share his life story—and the supposedly curmudgeonly cobbler had transformed in front of me, revealing both hardship and humor, hurt and happiness. I left the shop that afternoon, the doorbell jingling behind me, feeling inspired by my new friend and by the power of a good question.

Kat Vellos, author of the book *We Should Get Together: The Secret to Cultivating Better Friendships*, is a big believer in this, too. "Most of our conversations never make it onto the freeway. They get parked on the on-ramp," she told me. "A good question takes you to a place where you feel known and understood and so does the other person. You both feel closer to each other and more alive when that conversation is over."

A blog post she wrote called "Alternatives to *How Are You?*" went viral in 2021, motivating her to launch the Better

Conversations Calendar with 365 prompts, one for each day of the year. Since then, Kat's annual calendars have helped thousands of people become more socially healthy through better conversation, hanging on walls in bedrooms and corporate offices, used by everyone from elementary school teachers to newlyweds and executives. One of her favorite questions is "What's in your heart and on your mind today?"

You may not want to walk up to a stranger and ask for their life story, but you can definitely ask better questions in your conversations with family, friends, coworkers, and neighbors to get to know them more meaningfully or deepen your relationship more quickly. Try Kat's question. Or try my favorite: "What's your rose, thorn, and bud this week?" A rose is something good that happened or something you are grateful for. A thorn is something that is challenging you. And a bud is something you are looking forward to.

You can also search for "conversation card deck" online to find numerous options that you can keep on your dining table or coffee table and draw from when you're gathered together. I've used them at dinner parties with friends, events for complete strangers, and even my wedding reception dinner.

Another way I've seen this done especially well was by my friend Justin. He invited twenty people to his apartment for Shabbat dinner. Many of the guests were not religious, and many didn't know anyone except Justin, myself included.

We sat around a long table. Justin went through the Jewish rituals, including reciting Kiddush and uncovering challah loaves, and then we began to eat. But instead of letting us chitchat with the people next to and across from us as we would normally do at a dinner party, Justin invited us to do things a little differently by playing the Curiosity Game: He would ask one person a question—any question. That person would answer with everyone listening, then ask someone else a question. And so on, until everyone at the table had both asked and answered. And so the group conversation began.

An hour and a half, many laughs, and even some tears later, we were no longer strangers. That simple structure, combined with people's unique questions, everyone's willingness to be open and vulnerable, and the personal stories we shared, created an atmosphere that felt holy.

At your next dinner party, why not try the Curiosity Game and see what happens? Here are some of Justin's favorite questions to start you off:

- What is something you were afraid of when you were younger, that you're no longer afraid of today?
- What is a big risk you took that has paid off?
- What are you most excited about these days?
- Who was the biggest influence on you when you were growing up?
- What was the most meaningful gift you've ever received and the most meaningful gift you've ever given?

VULNERABILITY: DIVULGE SELECTIVELY
Especially if your strategy is to Tone or Flex

When I was in high school, my parents were in the thick of a difficult divorce. Confiding in my friends about what I was going through would have been an emotionally healthy thing to do, giving me an outlet for the stress. It also would have been a *socially* healthy thing to do, giving my friends a chance to know me better and support me through a challenging time.

But I didn't confide in them. I didn't talk about it with anyone other than my siblings. As a result, I realize in retrospect, I alienated myself from the opportunity for deeper connection. Friends who genuinely cared about me had no clue that underneath smiling, bubbly Kasley, there was someone struggling in silence. I felt alone, when I didn't need to feel alone.

This changed when I moved away to attend university, saw an excellent therapist who helped me sort through the backlog of emotions, and slowly learned to open up more. But it took years of practice, and I was well into my mid-to-late twenties before I fully appreciated how important vulnerability is for relationship building.

In social science, this is known as *self-disclosure*. Research has shown that when you disclose information about yourself, such as thoughts, feelings, aspirations, or failures, others perceive you as more likable.[6] And the benefit goes both ways; you perceive the people you confide in more favorably, too. We like people who confide in us, and we like the people whom we confide in.

In a 2022 systematic review, researchers at the University of Cambridge reported that when adolescents self-disclose in person, they experience higher-quality relationships and greater well-being.[7] (I wish my teen self had known this!) Self-disclosure was less rewarding if done online unless the teens were highly anxious, in which case the digital buffer helped them get comfortable with being vulnerable so they could then do so face-to-face.

Of course, opening up has to be done selectively and thoughtfully, with people who are trustworthy and at moments that are appropriate. Pouring your heart out to anyone anytime could backfire. But I have often found that vulnerability is worth the risk. It opens up the possibility of greater relatability, trust, and emotional intimacy. It invites deeper connection.

GRATITUDE: SAY THANKS WITH SINCERITY
Especially if your strategy is to Stretch, Tone, or Flex

Studies have shown that gratitude plays a key role in both forming and maintaining relationships.[8] For instance, appreciative romantic partners feel closer to each other, more satisfied with their relationship, and more committed to staying together.[9] According to the "find, remind, and bind" theory, feeling and expressing appreciation requires paying attention to what's positive about other people.[10] This helps you *find* new candidates for close relationships, *remind* yourself of what you love about your current relationships, and *bind* yourself more closely to loved ones by making them feel valued.[11]

For this reason, Robert Emmons, a psychologist and professor at the University of California, Davis, and a leading expert on gratitude, calls it "a relationship-strengthening emotion."[12] According to his research, the list of benefits of thankfulness is long, including feeling less lonely and more outgoing, experiencing higher levels of joy and lower levels of pain, and having a stronger immune system—showing how the physical, mental, and social pillars reinforce each other and the overall health temple.

To strengthen your social muscles, think of someone in your life who you haven't spoken with in a while. Reflect on one thing you admire about them. Then tell them directly by sending a text or email, calling them on the phone, writing them a card or letter, or telling them in person the next time you see them. Even a simple text has been shown to result in greater feelings of connectedness and support.[13]

GENEROSITY: FEEL GOOD BY DOING GOOD
Especially if your strategy is to Stretch, Tone, or Flex

During the pandemic, researchers conducted a randomized controlled trial—the gold standard in research—with users of Nextdoor, a neighborhood networking app that is used by one-third of households in the US and over three hundred thousand neighborhoods in eleven countries.[14] Users in the US, UK, and Australia were randomly selected to participate in a challenge, not unlike my 108-day project, in which they would perform small acts of kindness for their neighbors over four weeks. These acts might be lending a listening ear, chatting over the fence, mowing a neighbor's lawn, or helping someone pick up groceries. After a month, those who did acts of kindness felt more connected than those who did not. Whereas one in ten of the givers experienced feelings of loneliness at the start of the challenge, only one in twenty did by the end.[15]

I like this study for two reasons. First, it shows that generosity doesn't just help the recipient as you might suspect; it also helps the giver. Other research has found this, too. Led by investigators at the University of Oxford, a systematic review and meta-analysis of studies with over four thousand participants confirmed that helpers are happier.[16] The same researchers did a follow-up experiment to test whether the benefits changed depending on who the recipient was.[17] When people did acts of kindness for seven days, the boost to their well-being was consistent regardless of whether their generosity targeted close relationships or complete strangers. The more kind acts, the happier they were.

Second, the gestures didn't need to be grandiose to have meaningful effects. Simply being friendly helped people feel measurably less lonely in the Nextdoor study. Similarly, in a study in which people spent $5 or $20 on either themselves or someone else, those who gave the money away experienced more joy. Even $5 made a difference.[18]

BOUNDARIES: CHOOSE YOUR GATHERING DIET
Especially if your strategy is to Rest

Priya Parker, author of *The Art of Gathering*, offers advice for how to decide whether or not to attend a social event through what she calls *intentional guesting*: "the act of choosing whether, why, and how one attends a gathering."[19]

First, she recommends paying attention to how you feel when you receive an invitation. Are you over-the-moon excited? Just meh? Instantly stressed and dreading it? This should help you identify whether that relationship, community, or activity is generally nourishing or draining to your social health. Second, Priya suggests evaluating your *gathering diet*: "the total mix and type and amount of gatherings you choose to host and guest over a specific period of time to nurture a connected and boundaried relational life." This might involve reflecting on how many and what kind of social activities would best serve you right now, based on whether you are a Butterfly, Wallflower, Firefly, or Evergreen. Third, Priya emphasizes the importance of making a decision and sticking to it with an enthusiastic yes or a decisive yet kind no.

Being intentional about what events you attend, decline, host, or don't host can transform your social health, just as choosing what foods to buy, cook, eat, or not can transform your physical health—for better or worse.

That said, sometimes it's impossible to avoid people or situations that aren't fulfilling. For example, you might be a parent who frequently has to attend kids' birthday parties or school events with other parents you don't particularly click with. Or you might have to collaborate with team members or clients at work who ruffle your feathers. In these instances, show up, be friendly, leave as soon as appropriate, and then counteract it with something (or someone) that replenishes your social health.

THE COMING SOCIAL WELLNESS INDUSTRY

You can use the previous suggestions on your own. But increasingly, if you want a little help strengthening your social muscles, you will be able to choose from a variety of options.

For comparison, as our collective understanding of what it means to be healthy broadened from physical to mental, and the idea of taking care of our minds in addition to our bodies became mainstream, mental health companies flooded the market. Today, the mental health industry is booming, valued at over $380 billion globally in 2020 and expected to surpass $530 billion by 2030.[20]

We are about to see a similar influx with social health.

The first sign is the growing number of companies that have launched in the past few years aiming to address the loneliness epidemic. Having developed a mobile app to help people deepen their relationships back in 2013 and advised executive leadership teams in this space more recently, I've taken a particular interest in technology solutions and tracked hundreds of start-ups. These include digital platforms to help isolated older adults build community and apps to help employees feel less lonely while working from home. I celebrate these entrepreneurs for applying their skills to such an important need. Outside technology, thousands of initiatives have launched across sectors and around the world in recent years.

Many more products and services are on the way to help people proactively cultivate social health as an asset and a resource, regardless of whether they feel lonely. Let's explore a few examples of what will be available to you in the future.

A GYM FOR SOCIAL FITNESS

In North America, there are countless places you can go if you want to work out your body, from high-energy gyms to tranquil yoga studios. But where can you go that's a dedicated space for exercising your social muscles? Community centers and social clubs come to mind, but they don't typically train you in how to be socially fit the way an exercise facility trains you to be physically fit.

I predict that over the next five years, we will see the rise of social fitness gyms for this purpose. They will offer classes and other opportunities for adults to make new friends, learn how to connect more meaningfully, and generally practice relational skills.

One example of a brick-and-mortar approach already doing this is Peoplehood. In 2023, the founders of SoulCycle— a popular fitness company that offers indoor cycling classes at locations across the US, Canada, and UK—opened a "modern community center" in New York City for people to try a "workout for your relationships." Peoplehood's signature hour-long sessions focus on guiding people to share openly and practice attentive listening with a group of strangers. Monthly membership costs $165 at the time of this writing and includes five in-person sessions and unlimited virtual sessions.

I have not yet tried Peoplehood, but in general I'm optimistic about dedicated places for people to practice social health. I hope that more will emerge for a range of budgets to be accessible to more people.

A PERSONAL TRAINER FOR HUMAN CONNECTION

You can hire a personal trainer if you want to get into better physical shape or meet with a therapist to improve your mental health. But who can you turn to if you want guidance for your social health?

Remember Kat Vellos, the author I mentioned earlier? She is one of the world's first connection coaches. Formerly a user experience researcher and designer for tech products, she decided to pivot and apply her skills to adult friendship instead, hoping to make relationships more "user friendly."

Kat provides one-on-one coaching for individuals and group coaching for members of her Connection Club, a dedicated community of adults looking to get better at friendship. Members gather as a group once per month for mini-workshops, open discussions, and dedicated time to plan and work on their connection goals with accountability and encouragement. In between gatherings, they stay connected through a private online forum where they can ask questions, share resources, and generally feel less alone on the journey of prioritizing social health.

Just as with social fitness gyms, I predict that you will see many more options for connection coaching in the next five years.

A PRESCRIPTION FOR COMMUNITY

Soon, you'll be able to turn to your doctor for help, too.

The practice of *social prescribing* is when a doctor or another healthcare professional refers a patient to resources for basic needs that fall outside the scope of typical medical care, like housing, transportation, employment, food access, and—

increasingly—connection. Financial workshops, job fairs, museum trips, community gardening, walking groups, and cooking classes are all examples of activities that might be "prescribed." If you were isolated or lonely, for instance, your primary care physician could connect you to a *link worker* (essentially a social worker) who would help you find local opportunities to Stretch, Rest, Tone, or Flex your social health.

In the UK, where 76 percent of family doctors report that multiple patients visit them as a result of loneliness each day, this practice is well established.[21] The UK's public healthcare system, the National Health Service, has made social prescribing a "key component" of its strategy and employs well over three thousand link workers.[22]

Soon, those living in the US, Canada, and other countries will have access to this kind of support as well. In 2023, a report from the World Health Organization and other partners highlighted twenty-four countries that were implementing social prescribing, ranging from Austria to Australia, Portugal to Poland, Italy to Iran, and Spain to Singapore.[23]

Research so far suggests that this is a promising way to improve social health. A 2021 systematic review of studies specifically looking at loneliness concluded that both patients and providers found social prescribing helpful.[24] For instance, patients who received social prescriptions felt less lonely and more socially connected and, as a result, decreased their use of primary care services, according to a study published in the *British Medical Journal*.[25] Daniel Morse, founding director of Social Prescribing USA, whose mission is to make social prescribing available to every American by 2035, told me, "When you take medication, there are often negative side effects. But when you have a social prescription, there are often positive ripple effects." Thinking back to chapter 1, remember that the overall health temple is strengthened by reinforcing the social health pillar.

As with social fitness gyms and connection coaches, expect your doctor to ask you about your social health in future visits. I predict this will become the norm in the next ten years.

There are many ways to strengthen your social muscles, whether your strategy is to Stretch, Rest, Tone, or Flex—and in the years to come, you will have an ecosystem of opportunities and support for that purpose.

As we'll explore in the next chapter, every step you take to improve your social health counts. Just as you don't need to run a full marathon and can simply go for a walk to reap physical health rewards, exercising your social muscles doesn't have to mean overhauling your life.

Chapter 6

Take One Small Step for You, One Giant Leap for Social Health

Too often we underestimate the power of a touch, a smile, a kind word, a listening ear, an honest compliment, or the smallest act of caring, all of which have the potential to turn a life around.

—Leo Buscaglia

For years, we were told that in order to get healthy, we needed to walk ten thousand steps per day. Some people rose to the challenge and hit those steps day in and day out, but for many others that number was intimidating. More recently, this advice has been debunked. A 2023 meta-analysis examined data on over two hundred twenty-six thousand participants and concluded that walking fewer than four thousand steps per day is enough to significantly reduce your risk of dying from any cause.[1]

If you follow that thread and look into research on how small amounts of movement affect physical health, you'll find that even little shifts lead to health benefits. For instance, if you spend most of your day sitting, taking a three-minute break every half hour to do jumping jacks, walk up stairs, or take as few as fifteen steps can improve your blood sugar control, according to one study.[2]

What these findings reveal for physical health also ring true for social health: simple actions can yield meaningful results. This is good news for several reasons. First, we don't risk overwhelming ourselves with the social health equivalent of ten thousand steps per day; you don't need to keep in touch with every person you meet or get involved with every parent group, professional association, or community group that tries to recruit you (unless you want to!). Second, we can be empowered knowing that the right steps, even when small, lead to giant leaps of progress.

THE SURPRISE OF KINDNESS

On a Friday morning in early September shortly before my fifteenth birthday, my mom dropped me off for my first day of grade ten. Swallowing my anxiety and clutching a small dictionary in my hands as if it were a lifeline, I walked into the center courtyard of my new high school, where a bulletin board listed classroom assignments for the thousand or so students.

I scanned for my name and found it, but I couldn't understand where it said to go. The sign was in French.

I looked down at my English–French dictionary and realized that it wouldn't be much help. Blinking back nervous tears, I looked back up and around the large oval courtyard, framed by imposing cement buildings and tall, thin cypress trees. Students milled about, exclaiming *"Coucou!"* when they reunited with friends and giving each other *bisous*—cheek-to-cheek kisses—three times, as is customary in Montpellier, the nearby city in the south of France.

Putting the language barrier aside, there was another problem: I didn't have any friends.

After a few minutes of my mind and heart racing while I stood awkwardly and wondered what to do, the school principal happened to walk by. I was the first foreigner to attend the school, so he personally had enrolled me a few weeks prior. Although he didn't speak English, he quickly deduced the situation, took me to one of the cement buildings, and indicated that I should wait there. I breathed a short-lived sigh of relief.

Around thirty students were waiting in the same spot. One group of girls in particular looked me up and down, taking in my long flowy skirt and curly blond hair that stood out like a sore thumb. They kept talking among themselves, occasionally shooting a scrutinizing glance my way.

A few months prior, my mom had asked me if I was open to living in another country for a year to experience a different culture. My parents were divorced and my siblings were much older, already in their twenties and thirties, so it would be just the two of us. Saying yes was easy; I was excited for an adventure abroad. Now came the hard part: navigating the social dynamics of high school when I didn't know anyone and couldn't speak or understand the language. Under the gaze of these girls, I wondered if I had made a terrible mistake.

The introductory day lasted a few hours, during which the teacher shared a lot of probably useful information and gave us a tour of the school—none of which I understood. When the other students raised their hands to ask or answer questions, I kept silent and tried to be invisible, terrified I would be called on.

Then something happened that allowed me to breathe a deeper sigh of relief and come back on Monday with a bit more confidence: someone spoke to me in English. A boy noticed my dictionary and asked me where I was from. Born in the Netherlands but having lived in France for many years, he was trilingual. He introduced himself and we chatted. I had made my first friend.

On Monday, the first full day of classes included an English lesson. The teacher was thrilled to have a native speaker for the other students to practice with and proceeded to ask me all kinds of questions, thankfully in English, in front of the class: where I was from in Canada, what it was like there, why I was here. With my peers' attention fixed on me, I tried to make a friendly first impression.

Then we moved into the main lesson of the day, which was sharing "favorites" with each other—our favorite foods, favorite animals, favorite flowers. I enjoyed the chance to talk to more people, but I still felt nervous. For the most part, they all knew each other already; I was the outsider, the newbie, the foreigner. When the bell rang for lunch, everyone stood up and started bustling out, back to talking among themselves in French.

My mind and heart raced again as I collected my things and headed for the door: Would I have to eat lunch alone?

As I was leaving the classroom, a girl with short brown

hair, a black leather jacket, and kind eyes walked up to me and introduced herself. She said something in French that I didn't understand, so she tried again in tentative English: "Yoo eet wizz us?" Her thick accent confused me at first, so she repeated more slowly and gestured to the other girls: "Yoo eet wizz us?" It dawned on me that she was inviting me to have lunch with them. "Yes!" I practically shouted, "I mean oui, merci!"

For the next hour, the group of girls who had eyed me up and down on the first day excitedly bombarded me with questions in a mix of French and broken English while we ate lunch together. The next day, they indicated for me to join them again. And the next day. And the next.

Two weeks later, on my birthday, I came to school to find several cards waiting for me on my desk, handmade out of construction paper and decorated with drawings and stickers of my favorite foods, favorite animals, favorite flowers.

One year later, the girls and our whole class threw me a surprise goodbye party before I flew back to Canada. By that point, they had helped me learn French, patiently answering my questions until I could do school assignments on my own—until I even dreamed in French. More important, they had become close friends. That night, we pulled mattresses out into the middle of the vineyard behind our friend's house and stayed up late to talk and watch the stars, sleeping briefly before being woken by the sunrise glimmering on dewdrops through the fog.

To this day, I keep their cards in a box of mementos—and some of those girls, now women in their thirties, are still my friends nearly two decades later. Two of them traveled to the US to attend my wedding. I exchange updates and photos over WhatsApp with others. We may not see each other as often as we'd like, but our memories together and the bonds we formed over the course of that year will always connect us.

REACH OUT

The boy asking me where I was from, the girl inviting me to lunch, others leaving handmade birthday cards on my desk—these simple gestures of kindness sparked enduring friendships, fueled my social health during my year in France, and have made me appreciate the power of reaching out to this day. The fact that my peers welcomed and included me meant the world to me, especially given how nervous I was as a foreigner and how impressionable I was as a teenager.

Every day, kids eat lunch alone. In the US, one in five adolescents aged twelve to seventeen report doing so often.[3] A study of over one million teenagers in thirty-seven countries around the world found that the number of students who felt lonely at school nearly doubled between 2012 and 2018.[4] Whereas 17 percent of Baby Boomers grew up feeling lonely at least once per week, 39 percent of Gen Zers do—including 12 percent who say they feel lonely every single day.[5]

Feeling outcast isn't just hurtful in the moment; it can do lasting damage. A five-decade-long study in the UK tracked nearly eight thousand participants from childhood to their fifties.[6] Those who had been bullied as kids were less likely to have a partner or spouse, had trouble making and keeping friends, and had less social support available to them. Adolescence is a critical phase for developing social skills and forming one's identity, which means it can also be a time of particular vulnerability to social health threats.[7] Even one instance of peer rejection can be enough to cause significant distress.[8]

How much of this pain might be alleviated starting with one simple gesture of outreach?

YOU UNDERESTIMATE YOUR POWER

You are a superhero. Whether in the cafeteria, at a bar, or at the office, your ability to reach out and connect with someone—and in doing so bolster both their and your social health—is a superpower. Yet most people don't realize how much their simple actions mean to others.

In a 2023 paper published in the *Journal of Personality and Social Psychology*, researchers described a series of experiments in which they tested the effects of outreach, which could be as simple as sending a brief message to check in with someone and say, "I'm thinking of you." Whether to loved ones or casual acquaintances, the initiators (i.e., those who reached out) consistently and significantly underestimated how much the responders (i.e., those who were reached out to) would appreciate the gesture.[9]

People enjoy hearing from you more than you think.

Similarly, researchers at the University of Chicago found that when people sent a supportive email to someone who they knew was going through a tough time, they underestimated how positively the recipient would feel, overestimated how awkward the recipient would feel, and underrated how warmly and competently their email would be perceived.[10] Studies have found this same effect for random acts of kindness (such as giving away cups of hot chocolate at a park)[11] and expressions of gratitude (such as writing a letter to let someone know you appreciate them).[12]

The mismatch between how much impact you *think* your

outreach will have and how much impact your outreach *actually* has may make you reluctant to reach out in the first place—a misguided fear that could inhibit you from having a mutually meaningful interaction that furthers your relationship.

This is especially true given the principle *It Takes Two to Tango*. If you tend to rely on your friends and family to initiate, I challenge you to reciprocate more. On the other hand, if you are always the one who reaches out in a given relationship, ask yourself why. Is that person simply going through a busy time in their life? Do they have different preferences for the frequency of connection—maybe they're a Wallflower or Firefly, whereas you're a Butterfly or Evergreen? Or is the relationship not mutual in the way that you deserve?

Whether you want to Stretch, Tone, or Flex your social muscles, make a ritual of reaching out, and appreciate it when others reach out to you. It truly is a superpower. You don't need to wear a cape—you just need to wield your eyes and words, one interaction at a time.

THE RIPPLE EFFECTS OF CONNECTION

Growing up in Los Angeles, Darlene made some choices that led to serious consequences. "When I was sixteen, I was incarcerated," she shared with me. "I know firsthand how much isolation affects our social and mental health."

She also knows firsthand how incarceration affects families. Today, Darlene is a mom to three children whose dad is serving a long sentence. The strict rules in visiting rooms prevent her kids from hugging their dad or sitting closely with him for more than a few minutes. But this was even worse during the pandemic, when visiting rooms in prisons were closed to avoid spreading COVID-19.

In conversations with her daughter during that time, Darlene realized how hard the separation was for her and her siblings. Not only could they not see their dad, but they also had to stay home from school and couldn't hang out with friends. "That took a toll on them. It made me think about all the other children who were experiencing the same thing that my kids were. Children want to feel connected to their parents, no matter the circumstances."

When pandemic restrictions were lifted, Darlene vowed to give local youths and families the chance to come together. Social Health Labs awarded her a $1,000 microgrant in 2021 to organize a gathering for kids and for their parents who had recently been released from prison and were living in transitional homes before reintegrating into society. Transitional homes, too, had been closed to visitors until recently, so this would be one of the first times that many families were reuniting. Some parents would be meeting their kids, who had been born during their incarceration, for the very first time.

When Darlene shared the idea and news of the microgrant with others in the community, excitement grew. "It became bigger than I had imagined!" One organization donated a venue with a pool for the event; another donated sneakers for kids to take home with them. Darlene got supplies for people to paint, make T-shirts, and barbecue hamburgers. She called the event No Estás Solo—Spanish for You Are Not Alone.

On the day of No Estás Solo, forty families showed up. "It was such a beautiful day of bonding. I didn't get to take a lot of photos because I was busy hosting everybody, but also, these were moments that you couldn't really capture in a photo." Darlene teared up, remembering the interactions. "It makes me emotional thinking about it because all people want is connection. People who experience incarceration have this challenge to reconnect with their families. They have stigma that's wrapped around them. Sometimes all they want to do is build relationships with the people they feel they've wronged and the community they feel they've harmed.

"When we open the door to connection," she continued, "the possibilities are limitless. It helps individuals heal. It helps our children heal. Children's voices are not heard when their parents are incarcerated, so providing the space for them acknowledged that they weren't alone in the situation and they are not forgotten. They're valued. Their community and their families do love them and think about them."

The impact of Darlene's gathering transcends one happy afternoon. The event was so well received, people kept asking Darlene when she was going to host another. So she did. And her impact doesn't stop there. "I believe that when we build healthy relationships with our family, it helps reduce recidivism. And that helps our children because they get to grow up with their parents with them. That can break generational cycles."

I'm inspired by Darlene because she listened to her daughter, channeled her own painful experiences, galvanized her community, and organically grew opportunities for healing through connection. Recalling the Greek temple analogy in chapter 1, the interactions that day helped families begin rebuilding their social pillars at a challenging time of transition—and the ripple effects may benefit generations to come.

YOU JUST MIGHT SAVE A LIFE

Ethan Wall was a varsity basketball player and star athlete in a small rural town in Washington State. But when he came down with an illness that kept him homebound for multiple weeks, he did not receive a single phone call, text message, or visit from a friend. He felt completely cut off from his peers.

"It wasn't that the other kids didn't care," his older brother Luke told me. "It was just 'out of sight, out of mind.'" Ethan's isolation took him to a dark place quickly, leading to depression and suicidal ideation.

Their mom, Kristin, was dismayed by the lack of support from his peers and wondered, "How long does it take someone to write a text to say they care and press Send? Only seven seconds!" That experience led Kristin to create Only7Seconds (O7S), a nonprofit that seeks to teach empathy, compassion, and social skills to youths, as well to as inspire them with how simple it can be to connect meaningfully and make a difference in someone's life.

Thankfully, with family and professional support, Ethan made it through that period of darkness and is now a thriving adult, happily married. But others like him were not so lucky. A few years later, two boys who lived nearby passed away from suicide within two weeks of each other. Their deaths devastated the community—and galvanized the Wall family.

Within a month, the O7S website got over thirty thousand views. As word spread, more than thirty school districts around the country reached out asking for resources. The Walls, who until that point had been working on the nonprofit around the kitchen table in their spare time, realized they had to buckle down.

In 2021, Luke quit his job and took the reins. He gathered a dozen experts with different perspectives, including mental health professionals, educators, and students, for a weekend intensive to start developing the long-term strategy. They focused first on a campaign and podcast to raise awareness and a classroom course to move the needle. The Connection Curriculum they developed consists of a series of sessions focused on personal connections, empathy lessons, and connection challenges.

For personal connections, students visualize themselves at the center of connection circles. The smallest circle is for closest relationships. The next is for family and friends. And so on, out to casual acquaintances. Students reflect on whom they currently count in each circle, as well as whom they would like to add—a different approach to the worksheet you filled out in chapter 2 to evaluate your social health.

For empathy lessons, students learn to understand other people's perspectives and get inspired by watching video interviews with people who have undergone personal transformations. They hear from people like Mario, a sophomore in college who immigrated from Mexico, lost his mom at a young age, and was diagnosed with depression. Or Mariah, a high school junior in an abusive family who turned to bullying others. After each story, students share reflections in small groups.

For connection challenges, one week they might have to do an act of kindness in their community, such as expressing gratitude to a family member, posting something positive online, or helping out a stranger. Another week, the challenge might be writing letters to their future selves, with answers to prompts like "What are some ways you connect with yourself?" and "Who is someone you look forward to seeing every day and why?"

Luke and O7S, which quickly grew to a full-time team, started testing the Connection Curriculum in grades six through twelve at nine schools. The schools ranged from rural to urban, small to big, nearby to abroad. The results were encouraging. Based on assessments before and after participating, three-quarters of students felt less lonely.

"One of the biggest pieces of feedback we get from students is how impactful it is to hear stories that are both very similar to and very different from what they have gone through," Luke told me. "Kids will say, 'I thought I was the only one who experienced depression or lost a parent.' They realize they're not alone in their grief and struggles." Moreover, the opportunity to open up to each other when discussing the videos helped deepen their relationships at school.

Unexpectedly, the program also seemed to benefit the teachers who administered it—even more so than the students: nearly 85 percent reported feeling less lonely themselves. Luke believes this may be summed up by the Latin proverb *docendo discimus*: by teaching we learn.

At the time of this writing, I serve on the organization's Scientific Advisory Board, and O7S is gearing up to launch the next iteration of the curriculum, refining the lessons on the basis of insights from the pilot program and expanding to more schools throughout the US and internationally. As it grows, the ethos at the heart of all O7S does always comes back down to its name: Only7Seconds.

That's all the time it takes to reach out and show someone you care.

EXERCISES FOR SOCIAL FITNESS

It's time to put your superpower into action. Reach out by complimenting a stranger, inviting a friend to lunch, or introducing yourself to a new coworker. You could reach out to someone new if you want to Stretch or someone you are already close to if you want to Tone or Flex. As the research shows, the gesture doesn't have to be big to be effective—and it might blossom into a new friendship, deepen an existing relationship, or set off powerful ripple effects.

Or it might just make you feel a little happier today. Here are three evidence-based ideas to try.

TALK FOR TEN

As part of a randomized controlled study, adults aged 27 to 101 years who were homebound due to disability or health issues received ten-minute phone calls a few times per week from people who actively listened and asked questions to thoughtfully engage in conversation.[13] After four weeks, the recipients reported feeling significantly less lonely, less depressed, and less anxious.

There are two steps you can take inspired by this study. First, if you know someone who is homebound, like a neighbor or relative, call them to check in and chat, even briefly. Second, your loved ones would likely appreciate a call from you regardless of whether they are homebound or not—and I'll bet you would enjoy it, too. Pick a friend or family member you haven't spoken with lately and talk with them for ten minutes.

EAT TOGETHER

In the US, only 38 percent of Gen Zers and 46 percent of Millennials say they grew up having daily meals with their families, compared with 59 percent of Gen Xers, 76 percent of Baby Boomers, and 84 percent of the Silent Generation.[14] That's a clear decline over time in how often families sit down and eat together.

Anne Fishel, who directs the Family and Couples Therapy Program at Massachusetts General Hospital and teaches at Harvard Medical School, cofounded the Family Dinner Project to encourage more parents to make mealtime a priority. "As a family therapist, I often have the impulse to tell families to go home and have dinner together rather than spending an hour with me," she has written, because "dinner is the most reliable way for families to connect and find out what's going on with each other."[15]

Make family meals a priority. And if you don't have kids or don't live near your parents, for instance, try a "family" dinner tradition with friends, neighbors, or your partner at least once a week.

INTRODUCE YOURSELF

Marcus had heard there was a new person in the building. He lived in a small, ornate Victorian on top of a hill in San Francisco, with just twelve units on three floors and a single staircase, no elevator. So when he was walking down the stairs one morning and encountered a woman walking up whom he hadn't seen before, he introduced himself. She smiled and they chatted for a few minutes before going their separate ways.

He couldn't stop thinking about her all day, so the next morning he left a bottle of wine and a card outside her door, welcoming her to the building and the neighborhood. Five years later, Marcus married her.

That woman was me.

Introduce yourself to your neighbors. You never know where it might lead.

WHAT IF EVEN SMALL STEPS FEEL DAUNTING?

I want to acknowledge that small steps can seem like giant leaps if you struggle with social anxiety, if you feel shy or self-conscious, if you have a disability that makes social interaction especially challenging, if past negative experiences left you feeling rejected or excluded by peers, if you've gone through a recent life change that disrupted your usual social patterns, if you haven't exercised your social muscles in a while, or for any other of myriad possible reasons.

Reaching out might come more naturally to you if your style is Butterfly or Evergreen because you are more extroverted and comfortable with a high frequency of interaction. If you are a Wallflower or Firefly, taking the initiative to connect out of the blue might feel awkward at first—just as your body is particularly sore the first few times you try a new workout. Know that with practice, it will get easier—and it's likely to feel better than you expect. If you recall from chapter 3, we can all benefit from stepping outside our usual connection preferences and habits to try something new.

Honestly? I doubt there is or has ever been a human on Earth who didn't find connection difficult at some point. I still do sometimes. It takes courage to reach out and try to connect, just as it takes courage to date and try to find love. Sometimes it will go well; sometimes it won't.

But it is absolutely worthwhile. Putting effort into your social health is an act of love to yourself—a way you can care for and advocate for *you*. You can't always rely on other people to initiate, waiting passively for mutual, meaningful connection to fall in your lap. You have choices. You have agency. And there are opportunities all around you, if you open yourself to them.

The advice I give to those for whom small steps feel daunting is to look for the right opportunities. Is talking on the phone more enjoyable for you than meeting in a loud public space? Does doing an activity with someone else, like hiking or touring an art gallery, make it easier for you to engage in conversation than sitting face-to-face? The trick is determining which ways of engaging with people are right for you.

In the next chapter, we'll explore a powerful mindset that can help you do exactly that.

Chapter 7

Think Like a Scientist, Even If You're Not One

One knows from daily life that one exists for other people—first of all for those upon whose smiles and well-being our own happiness is wholly dependent, and then for the many, unknown to us, to whose destinies we are bound.

—Albert Einstein

Figuring out what your optimal social health looks like and how to cultivate it takes an open mind, a sincere interest in your relationships and communities, and a willingness to test new approaches.

That final part—testing new approaches—is the last piece of the puzzle when it comes to putting the theory of social health into practice. You have learned why it is critical to your well-being, seeing the social pillar as foundational to your overall health temple, and you have learned various methods for Stretching, Resting, Toning, and Flexing. But how exactly do you know which works for you? And how can you navigate inevitable setbacks?

This is where a mindset of experimentation comes into play.

As a social scientist by training, I like to experiment not only in my work but also in my personal life—including with my social health. That means coming up with hypotheses, testing them, and then refining my ideas and actions on the basis of the results.

By now, you've gotten a sense of some of the experiments I've done to foster connection, from doing acts of kindness for 108 days in a row to walking up to a complete stranger in a shoe repair shop and asking for his life story. When applying this mindset to my social health, it didn't take formal data collection or analyses to understand the outcome of my actions.

Even if you've never laid eyes on a research paper and haven't calculated statistics since high school math class, there are certain qualities that scientists possess that may help you, too, when exercising your social muscles. No lab coat required.

A GOOD SCIENTIST IS CURIOUS

Rowan found himself in need of experimentation when he went through a major life change that left him feeling disconnected. In his mid-thirties, he moved back to his hometown, Atlanta, to start his dream job. By day, he enjoyed work. But on nights and weekends, he felt unfulfilled—eating meals alone more often than not, spending hours at the gym to fill the time.

He didn't know how to get out of his rut until he read one of my articles and emailed me. In doing so, Rowan demonstrated curiosity and a willingness to learn and try new things—traits of a good scientist—so I challenged him to a monthlong experiment.

First, we talked through the three-step method of evaluating his social health, starting with identifying his sources, reflecting on how mutually and meaningfully connected he felt to each, and deciding what his overall strategy should be.

His closest source until recently had been his girlfriend of three years, until she broke up with him. Not only was he reeling from the loss of the woman he envisioned marrying, but he also had to adjust to the change in his social patterns. Whereas she was a Butterfly, he was a Wallflower, so he had largely relied on her to organize outings. Without her influence, Rowan felt noticeably more alone.

His family sources included his parents and sister, all of whom lived nearby in Atlanta, so he started seeing them once or twice per month for lunch or dinner. However, Rowan's family relationships were complicated, and spending time with them sometimes left him feeling drained. He worried about his parents getting older and more dependent, and his sister seemed to have her life all figured out despite being younger, which he admitted left him feeling behind.

Rowan's next sources were a handful of close friends who lived elsewhere, with whom he spoke on the phone a couple of times each month. These relationships were positive and supportive—they were people he could reach out to when he was feeling down. But it was harder to spend time with them now that he lived farther away and now that several had gotten married and started having kids. Meanwhile in Atlanta, most of the people he knew from childhood and college had moved away, except for one casual friend named Jeff and a few acquaintances.

At work, Rowan was just starting to get to know his coworkers. There was one in particular named Linden whom he immediately got along with.

Overall, he didn't yet have as many sources as he wanted in Atlanta, and the sources he did have there were not as strong as he would like. The pandemic had left Rowan feeling rusty about socializing with new people, and the breakup had rattled his self-confidence—compounding his already introverted nature and making social health seem elusive. Thinking back to the 5–3–1 guideline we discussed in chapter 3, he was not consistently connecting with five different people per week and wanted to, he *did* have three close relationships but not nearby, and he liked the goal of at least one hour of quality connection each day on weekends, though not necessarily on weekdays after a long day of work.

Given this, Rowan decided his strategy was to Stretch—to spend less time alone, make new friends, and find a sense of community in his new home.

KNOW YOU'RE NOT ALONE

A lot of men feel similarly to Rowan—and there's no shame in it. Remember: *What Goes Down Will Come Up*. We all experience highs and lows in our social lives.

The decline in friendships in recent decades seems to have hit men harder than women. Between 1990 and 2021, the percentage of men in the US who reported having no close friends rose from 3 percent to 15 percent. In the same time period, those who reported having at least five close friends dropped from 68 percent to 41 percent.[1] A survey in the UK revealed that the average age of men who felt isolated was thirty-five, and both moving and going through a breakup were among the top reasons.[2] No wonder Rowan was feeling the way he did.

To counter this overall trend, the small town of Goolwa in South Australia set up a shed for men. From the outside, it looked like an unassuming workshop or storage unit. But inside, you might find one man fixing a broken lawn mower, someone else building a table, and others sitting together and drinking coffee. Today, more than fifty thousand men frequent more than one thousand two hundred sheds across Australia; there are more men's sheds than McDonald's restaurants there. The movement has spread to other countries, too, including the US, Ireland, Kenya, and South Africa.

"Many men, especially after retirement, find themselves alone, often living in isolation and needing to connect with their community and find new purpose but aren't sure how. Others just want to learn a new skill or revisit old ones," explains the Australian Men's Shed Association on its website. "Becoming a member of a Men's Shed provides a safe and busy environment where men can find many of these things in an atmosphere of old-fashioned mateship." (I had to look up *mateship*; it's an Australian term for camaraderie.) New members of any age and background are welcome to join.

Men's sheds promote physical, mental, and social health, often without members even realizing it—which some describe as "health by stealth." For instance, in a 2022 systematic review, researchers in Germany reported that men who frequented the sheds gained a sense of belonging, were more physically active, and enjoyed greater well-being.[3]

Knowing how common Rowan's experience is and how

many opportunities like men's sheds there are, I suggested that he think like a scientist and try at least one new kind of social activity each week for one month to see which relationships or communities feel right. As his first step to Stretch his social muscles, Rowan decided to take an improv workshop. I was surprised that he chose such an outgoing activity, given how he was feeling, but that's exactly what made it such a great idea— sometimes we all need to do something that knocks us out of the headspace we're stuck in.

Improv was a success. Being playful loosened him up, and he had so much fun that he ended up signing up for an ongoing class. "A highlight was that I met a couple new people who live near me," Rowan shared. "One invited me to play basketball with him, and we exchanged contact info." He had made his first new friend.

Thanks to Rowan's curiosity and openness, the experiment was off to a good start.

A GOOD SCIENTIST IS OBJECTIVE

As I explained with the principle *To Each Their Own,* social health is subjective. Only you can determine how connected you feel, and the way you go about connecting is a matter of personal preference.

But if you are trying to establish new sources and something doesn't work, it's best to be more objective. This means not taking the outcome too personally. For example, if you go to an event run by a group you're interested in joining, but you don't enjoy it that much, move on. Or if you meet up with a potential new friend and find that you don't really click with them—or that they don't seem that interested in you—shrug it off.

Unless you're rude, it's unlikely that the interactions went awry because something is wrong with you. It's more likely that the person or the group is simply not the right fit.

That's not always easy, I know. Coming away from an interaction feeling rejected, feeling like you don't belong, or just feeling unfulfilled without necessarily being able to put a finger on why—these feel deeply personal. But I invite you to think like a scientist: see each negative social experience as a data point that reveals an insight and points you in a better direction.

For his next step, Rowan went to a craft beer club social that he found online on Meetup. The event description said that anyone who liked craft beer could come to socialize and hang out; the group met monthly at different breweries and bars around the city. He was nervous when he showed up on a Friday after work, ordered a beer, and introduced himself. He relaxed once he started talking with people in the group and found them welcoming. But he nonetheless left that night feeling unsatisfied—aside from enjoying beer, he didn't really click with the people he spoke to.

When we talked on the phone the next day, I could hear the disappointment in his voice. Instead of comforting him, I exclaimed, "Congrats!" He gave a confused laugh, so I reiterated: "Seriously, that's a helpful data point. That particular community may not be the right fit for you, so you can move on to the next. Frankly, the worse your social activities go, the greater clarity you'll have about what you're looking for—plus, the better stories you'll have to share with me, and the more we can laugh it off together. Some will go well, some won't, and that's not a reflection on you. That's a normal part of the process."

A good scientist is committed to finding the truth by conducting many studies. Some fail. Some yield significant results. Science is an iterative process of trial and error. So it is with finding relationships and communities that are meaningful to you.

Of course, you have to show up and put in your best effort. But getting attached to the result of any one interaction or activity in particular isn't helpful. There are too many factors outside your control—like, in Rowan's case, whether the other people who showed up to the craft beer social had other similarities they could bond over. Rowan was better off seeing this experience as one of many data points he was going to collect, rather than a definitive sign about his ability to find a new community where he belonged.

Plus, it had been a big step forward in challenging his inner Wallflower.

ASSUME PEOPLE LIKE YOU

In a 2018 study, researchers from Cornell, Harvard, and Yale Universities and the University of Essex paired up strangers and instructed them to have five-minute conversations.[4] Afterward, they pulled each individual aside and privately asked how much they liked the other person and how much they thought the other person liked them.

The researchers found that participants consistently and significantly underestimated how much others enjoyed their company. Yet when neutral observers watched recordings of these conversations later on, they could reliably tell when someone liked the other person. In other words, it was obvious to outsiders, but not to the people in the interaction, how much they hit it off with the other person. Social psychologists call this discrepancy between how you think people perceive you and how they actually perceive you the *liking gap*.

It means that people probably like you more than you realize.

Marisa G. Franco, a psychologist and author of *Platonic: How the Science of Attachment Can Help You Make—and Keep—Friends*, offers a straightforward solution: "Assume people like you."[5] This mindset not only is more accurate but also can influence your behaviors for the better. "It's a self-fulfilling prophecy. Research actually finds that we're warmer and more engaged when we make this assumption." In turn, people perceive you as even more likable—and the relationship can more easily flourish.

For Rowan's next step, he decided to get lunch with Linden, the person at work who had stood out to him. Linden worked on a different team, but they had met at an office mixer during Rowan's first week at work and had quite a bit in common—both had previously lived in New York, liked running, and were passionate about their field. The next time Rowan ran into Linden at the office, though, and tried striking up a conversation, Linden seemed disinterested. Rowan wasn't sure what to make of it and felt awkward—as if he were trying to ask a woman out on a date—so he didn't mention lunch.

It was possible that Linden was disinterested—or maybe he was distracted because he was running late for a meeting. Maybe he was stressed about an upcoming deadline. Maybe he was tired because he had a sick kid at home who had kept him up the night before. There were so many possible explanations. "Assume he likes you," I suggested to Rowan, echoing Marisa's advice, "and ask him to lunch next time you see him."

Rowan did. Linden accepted. They had a great conversation, and Linden invited Rowan to a barbecue he was hosting the following weekend.

A GOOD SCIENTIST IS PERSISTENT

Scientists may attempt many failed experiments before finding noteworthy results. Persistence is part of the process. So it is when experimenting with social health. Coming back to the principle *What Goes Down Will Come Up,* social health ebbs and flows just as physical and mental health do. To endure the lows so that you can enjoy the highs requires not giving up, being patient, and continuing to experiment.

KEEP LOOKING UNTIL YOU FIND YOUR PEOPLE

In the final week, Rowan reached out to Jeff, the friend from college who was still living in Atlanta. They had lost touch over the years, but they had good memories of being students together. The two met for dinner.

Rowan reported that he enjoyed it overall, but it prompted him to reflect on what kind of friendship he was seeking. Thinking back to the principle *Quality over Quantity,* he realized he didn't want *many* friends as much as he wanted *good* friends.

After reminiscing about college days, Rowan found that he and Jeff no longer had much in common. As well, Jeff had looked at his phone multiple times during dinner, which Rowan found himself interpreting as a sign that Jeff wasn't having a good time. We again discussed the liking gap and how there could be alternative explanations—maybe Jeff did that with everyone, or maybe there was something going on that he needed to respond to.

At the same time, we discussed that he could set the bar higher for close friendships. If it was important to Rowan to not have to constantly question and second-guess whether someone liked him, he should probably find people who spoke his friendship language loudly and clearly—people who gave him their full attention during dinner, for example. Jeff didn't seem compatible in this way, and that was okay. They didn't need to become best friends.

We should all have high standards when it comes to whom we spend time with.

By the end of his one-month experiment, Rowan had successfully made two new friends—one at the improv workshop and one being Linden from work. He had figured out that the craft brew club was not the right community for him and that having friends who were present and engaged was important to him. He had also gained confidence and felt more optimistic overall. These were meaningful steps forward in his strategy to Stretch.

At the same time, his social health was—and is—a work in progress. Developing the new friendships would take time, and Rowan was still mourning his breakup and figuring out how to be around family in a way that felt nourishing. Setting up a personal experiment helped him to be intentional about connection, to prioritize it despite being busy settling into his new job and home, and to overcome the hurdle of feeling lonely and blue. The mindset would help him keep being curious, objective, and persistent as he exercised his social muscles going forward.

How might you set up an experiment to Stretch, Rest, Tone, or Flex over the next month? What is your equivalent to trying an improv workshop or inviting a coworker to lunch?

KEEP GOING UNTIL YOU FEEL CONNECTED

When Richard was growing up, he didn't have many friends. He was an only child and naturally shy. His parents worked hard to build their new life in Calgary, Canada, having immigrated from Vietnam shortly before he was born. Social skills like how to make friends or communicate effectively weren't modeled at home, nor taught in school, so Richard turned to television shows, movies, and books for guidance. However, those portrayed main characters hanging out with their best friends, which didn't match his reality. "For a long time, I thought I must be doing something wrong," he confessed to me.

When Richard began his undergraduate degree at a small university in a rural town a couple of hours' drive from home, he again felt lonely—until he began interviewing students and faculty for a project inspired by *Humans of New York*, the blog and book of portraits and interviews with strangers on the streets of New York City started by the photographer Brandon Stanton in 2010. (If you haven't seen it before, it's worth checking out as a beautiful way to empathize with people from all walks of life.)

In his conversations, Richard realized that he was making friends by being curious about their lives and asking questions that went beyond small talk. To his surprise, many of the older students, who he assumed had it all figured out, expressed how they had felt out of place and had a hard time making friends in their first year.

"That's when it clicked," he recalled. "I realized I wasn't alone in feeling lonely. There wasn't something wrong with me. It's just that this topic isn't talked about much, so people feel a sense of stigma and shame. If it was normalized, I think I wouldn't have suffered as much."

Richard first read about the idea of social health in one of my articles, and it immediately resonated with him. "I wish social health had been taught to me from a young age and modeled to me. I wish I hadn't had all these misconceptions, like thinking I should have one best friend. I realized later on that it's unhealthy for me to expect any one person to fulfill all my social needs. I can feel fulfilled by having different groups of friends and communities for all my interests."

He went on: "I know that at one point, mental health was not a widely discussed topic. Now if social health becomes part of our vocabulary, too, with education and awareness, I think it will alleviate a lot of these challenges. People end up blaming themselves for what they think is their own social incompetence, and that leads them to keep to themselves because they don't want to put themselves out there and risk being vulnerable or getting hurt. It's a negative cycle that they get stuck in—that I got stuck in. In fact, rejection is part of the process. You're not going to get along with everyone, and that's okay. You still have self-worth."

In 2021, Richard graduated a much more confident and socially healthy version of himself than when he first arrived on campus, having Stretched and Toned his social muscles to free his inner Firefly. Two years later, Richard returned to that same campus, this time to help new students who might be feeling like he had. The university hired him to implement a school-wide strategy that he had pitched them to create systems and spaces that foster social health among students.

"I've learned that partly it's on individuals to put ourselves out there and put in the effort, but partly it's not," he explained. "If this is never taught, whether through your upbringing from your parents or through school from your teachers, then it's not *really* your fault."

Richard's first task with the university was coordinating shared spaces on campus called REC Rooms, with ping-pong tables, giant chess sets, and other activities, for students to hang out and connect through play. In a survey, one student shared, "I was very much alone for the first month I was here.

But I made my first group of friends at the REC Room and continue to hang out with them regularly." Next, Richard educated the campus community through events and presentations. "Most people don't know what social health is when I bring up the term to them, just like I didn't until I read your articles. I want everyone to have this vocabulary." Finally, he tested various connection initiatives, such as putting QR codes on tables in high-traffic areas like food courts, which students could scan with their smartphones to access social health resources. One resource might be a list of conversation starters that go a little deeper than "How are you?"

"I sort of see the whole campus as my lab," Richard said. "I'm running experiments to see what might have an impact on the social health of students." He has since brought his connection initiatives and social health presentations to other universities and colleges, too.

Richard inspires me because he went from feeling disconnected in his youth to literally teaching social health. And if he can strengthen his social muscles—and help others do the same—by adopting a mindset of experimentation, so can you.

EXPERIMENT ACCORDING TO YOUR STYLE
How you experiment may differ based on whether you are a Butterfly, Wallflower, Firefly, or Evergreen.

Let's say your goal is to Tone (deepen your connections) and you are a Butterfly or Wallflower. Pick a friend you trust and try to go deeper using one of the suggestions in chapter 5. For example, you could try having a deeper conversation by asking a question like "What's in your heart and on your mind today?" or "What's your rose, thorn, and bud this week?" Then answer it in return, opening up with something more personal than you normally would. Reflect afterward: Did your friend receive it well and reciprocate? Do you feel closer to them? Or do you have a vulnerability hangover? If you're a Firefly or Evergreen, you might not need to experiment in this way because deeper connection comes more naturally to you.

Or let's say you're a Butterfly or an Evergreen and want to Rest (maintain or reduce your number of sources). In your case, choosing your gathering diet will be especially important. Maybe you decide, for the next month, to accept invitations to social events only from people you are very close to, declining any that come from looser ties and instead spending that time reconnecting with yourself. After a month, recalibrate. Do you feel more balanced? Or did you find yourself missing more casual interaction?

Go back to the worksheet you filled out in chapter 2 and write down a few ways that you can experiment in the next week or month, given your overall strategy. Whatever your style, remember to stay curious, objective, and persistent.

WHEN TO BE LESS LIKE A SCIENTIST AND MORE LIKE A HUMAN

I have a confession. Sometimes when I take off my academic hat—the one I got from working as a researcher and spending time in the ivory tower of universities—and put on my regular human hat, I find that parts of the scientific way of seeing the world aren't helpful outside of studies. Certain qualities that are assets in research can be crippling in everyday life. So here are a few to avoid as you experiment with your social health.

DON'T BE TOO CRITICAL

When training as a social scientist, I learned to be skeptical and scrutinizing, searching for overlooked nuances and shortcomings to critique in every study. This is helpful for advancing research but *not* helpful in relationships or on your journey to finding what social routines and communities are right for your socially healthy lifestyle. Instead, be playful and optimistic. Social health is fun! There's nothing better than spending time with people you adore, who adore you in return.

DON'T BE TOO RATIONAL

Logic and quantitative data are core to science. But with human connection, pay attention to how you *feel*. Definitely assess the outcomes of your experimentation and consider factors like whether the connection feels mutual (*It Takes Two to Tango*). But in doing so, prioritize what your gut tells you, even if it's hard to explain. You might be surprised by the people and groups you are drawn to when you listen to your heart rather than your brain. You might also be surprised by what repels you; remember that not all connection is good connection. Spending time and energy on people who don't feel right to you is not good for your social health.

DON'T BE TOO HARD ON YOURSELF

Many academics feel a lot of pressure to make scientific breakthroughs, publish regularly in prestigious journals, and achieve tenure—often leading to burnout.[6] As you experiment with your social health, be kind to yourself. Don't worry if you're too busy at work one week to connect with anyone other than coworkers. Don't beat yourself up if you need to prioritize other things for a few months and let your relationships fall to the wayside. We all do at times, myself included. Give yourself grace, and take care of your other needs as well. Social health is one pillar in the overall temple of your health and well-being; at times, it will be more important to focus on the others.

As we've explored in part II, the practice of social health entails making it a priority, learning to strengthen your social muscles, taking small steps that lead to big impact, and having a mindset of experimentation. Tying this all together and bringing it into the community you live in, the places you frequent in person and online, and the structures that make up the society around you is how you go from an idea to a way of life.

That brings us to part III.

Part III

AMPLIFY

Social Health as a Way of Life

Chapter 8

Build Community Where You Live

Each one of us matters, has a role to play, and makes a difference. Each one of us must take responsibility for our own lives, and above all, show respect and love for living things around us, especially each other.

—Jane Goodall

Having moved numerous times and lived in small towns and big cities in three countries, I've learned that the norms regarding how people connect are different in each place. My social health—and with it my physical and mental health—has been strongly influenced by how well I've been able to build friendships and community in each of the places I've lived.

Relocating so many times sparked my interest in how places affect social health. During my graduate work, I became fascinated by which design features in our buildings, neighborhoods, and cities either encourage or inhibit human connection. I was fortunate to collaborate with Ichiro Kawachi, a renowned social epidemiologist and professor at the Harvard T.H. Chan School of Public Health, to study this topic. I learned, for instance, that green spaces such as public parks, community gardens, and tree-lined streets help reduce loneliness, while neighborhoods that are walkable, with residential, commercial, and recreational properties close together, facilitate opportunities for interaction. We published a chapter in the second edition of the textbook *Making Healthy Places* for architects, civil engineers, urban planners, and other professionals to use these and other research insights in their work.

But what about you and me? What can we do in our own neighborhoods to bring people together? The best answers to these questions are found not in textbooks but in the world around us.

At nineteen years of age, I was lucky to return to France and spend six months in Paris for my studies. But as romantic as that sounds—and it was an enriching experience in many ways—it was also one of the most isolated times in my life. True to their reputation, Parisians didn't strike me as particularly warm. No one smiled on the metro. The waiters were brusque. Outside of classes, I struggled to meet people, make friends, and find a sense of community, despite speaking the language. My only interaction with a neighbor was when the one next door banged on the wall and yelled at me to turn down my music.

Fast-forward to 2022. I was deep into my work running Social Health Labs, as well as partnering with organizations to address loneliness as a public health issue and cultivate social health proactively and preventively as an asset and resource. I found myself asking a central question: What are models of communities that redefine health to include connection? Given that social health helps us live longer, healthier, and happier, where are examples of neighborhoods that are doing this well?

I heard that a group in Paris had banded together around *convivialité*—friendliness. Given my experience with the lack of friendliness there, I had to see it for myself. What I would find was a blueprint and vision for how individuals can band together to create a socially healthy community.

TO KNOW YOUR NEIGHBORS, START WITH HELLO

November in Paris was how I had always known Parisians to be: cold.

As I walked out of the metro in the 14th District on a November morning, a couple of miles south of the Seine River, I realized that I had not worn a thick enough coat to last long outside. I hurried into Café du Rendez-Vous and met Patrick Bernard, leader of the group that calls itself La République des Hyper Voisins—the Republic of Super Neighbors.

Patrick embodied *convivialité* long before we sat down together. His messages over email and WhatsApp leading up to my visit were warm and inviting, as was his presence now that we sat face-to-face—his face round, framed by graying hair, and decorated with equally round spectacles. We ordered breakfast, which in Paris means croissants, baguette, Nutella, coffee, and grapefruit juice (I also ordered eggs to lessen the culture shock to my stomach). Patrick began telling me the history of Super Neighbors.

A journalist for over twenty-five years, he had spent his career sharing information through articles. But in recent years, he had noted a change in the way information spreads. When his son, then a teenager, told him there was no need to pay for a newspaper when he could get all the news he needed online and on social media for free, Patrick realized that information was no longer valuable in the same way. So what was?

As he explored this curiosity further, he arrived at an answer that would ultimately inspire him to leave his job and dedicate himself to his community. Value in an age of passive, fleeting global consumption of information, he concluded, comes from the opposite: active, long-lasting local connection.

In April 2017, Patrick gathered five neighbors and proposed that instead of saying *"Bonjour"* a few times when they leave the house, the goal should be to say hello fifty times—to know enough people in the neighborhood to make that possible. To accomplish this, he proposed setting up a table on the street long enough for one thousand people to eat together and get to know each other.

The five neighbors laughed at the idea, deeming it impractical. But they nonetheless agreed with the underlying sentiment: there is value in knowing more neighbors. Their conceding was all he needed. Patrick became resolute.

Armed with his determination and a team of volunteers, who quickly grew from five to many as more people learned about the event and stepped up to help, Patrick brought his idea to fruition in September that same year. They set up tables and chairs stretching the length of Rue de l'Aude, a residential street in the heart of the 14th District, and sent out an open invitation to gather, share a meal, and connect. More than one thousand people came.

Since then, the Table d'Aude, as it is now known, has become an annual tradition, with a couple of exceptions during the height of pandemic lockdowns. It has spawned friendships, romances, and a sense of community for thousands of locals. The mayor of Paris has attended. The idea spread beyond France, including being replicated in Manhattan.

A sociologist who evaluated Super Neighbors concluded that the group successfully reduced social isolation, strengthened social ties, and improved resilience, not just through the Table d'Aude but also through ongoing events and programming.[1] Patrick told me that these benefits were clear when the pandemic hit. People who had met at the Table were quick to organize WhatsApp groups around various needs and interests, with hundreds of members communicating and supporting each other. The groups remained active and kept growing long after confinements ended.

Those groups leave a hint that Super Neighbors is about much more than a communal meal on the street once per year and saying hello fifty times when one leaves the house, although they do try to do that. ("We can't go back home if it's any less!" joked one of the neighbors I spoke with later.) Those are entry points into a more profound, ambitious change that they are endeavoring to bring about.

As we continued sipping our coffees and the café, nearly empty when we arrived, began to bustle with people, Patrick shared the longer-term vision. He described his current role as Ami du Quartier—Friend of the Neighborhood—connecting people, coordinating events, working full-time to advance this work. In the future, Super Neighbors envisions Friends of the Neighborhood throughout Paris, in every district, funded by the local government. The group intends to set up a school with certification programs to train new Friends of the Neighborhood in best practices, although each would tailor how they operate according to the unique needs and preferences of residents in their area.

Imagine that: one person in every neighborhood across the city responsible for improving social health locally. What might that look like where you live?

FROM ONE PERSON TO THOUSANDS OF CONNECTIONS

I swallowed my last bite of croissant just as Patrick looked at his watch and announced that we were running late. It was Saturday morning, and on Saturday mornings the Super Neighbors meet in the back corner of a particular local restaurant to drink coffee together and plan their activities. All are welcome, and different people drop in on different weekends, but the regulars consist of around a dozen older residents.

As we paid the waiter and began heading to the meeting, Patrick explained: "There are different spheres of involvement with Super Neighbors, and people participate how they can. We have the most active, which is mainly me and some older neighbors whom you'll meet shortly. They have the most free time, without jobs during the week or little kids to take care of on the weekends, so it makes sense. Then there are people who are active when they can be, volunteering at events and helping organize the WhatsApp groups."

We walked along a paved walkway in the middle of Avenue René-Coty, with tall trees and mature bushes separating us from the traffic on either side. Benches and chairs dotted the greenery, inviting passersby to pause on their promenade and reminding me of my graduate work studying the importance of shared spaces where people can connect outside of home or work.

"Then there are people who just show up and enjoy the events," Patrick continued. "Maybe they don't even know that an event is put on by Super Neighbors, but they benefit from it, and that's great. Then there are people who know about us but choose not to be involved, which is fine, too. Some people just want to live here and not be bothered—that's up to them. And finally, there are people who don't know about us, who we haven't reached yet."

Ascending a flight of stairs and turning a corner, we came to the street where the Table d'Aude is held each year. "Et voilà!" Patrick stopped so I could take it in. Modest yet quint-essentially Parisian, the cobblestone road was lined with lit-tle apartment buildings and occasional planter boxes, their shrubs and flowers beginning hibernation for winter. Pat-rick pointed out a tall mural painting of two trees and mice busying around—one sweeping leaves, another climbing a ladder—which Super Neighbors had commissioned from a local artist to brighten the wall of an affordable housing com-plex. The mural signified neighbors going about their days in the community.

Farther along, we passed a small communal garden—as big as the small Parisian street could accommodate. Translated, a sign next to two large compost boxes read, "We meet regularly with neighbors to garden, water, and maintain this place in joy and good humor. . . . Everyone is free to join us. . . . We gener-ally meet on Sundays in the late afternoon, depending on the weather."

I thought about how much I would have loved to participate in a communal garden as welcoming as this one, to meet more people and put down roots—literally—when I lived in Paris. But there hadn't been anything like this in my district. It occurred to me that the willingness to connect with neighbors, make new friends, and contribute to the community is probably more common than explicit opportunities to do so. Or perhaps I hadn't done a good job of trying to find those opportunities—or creating them myself. Over the course of investigating this topic and implementing solutions with partners across sectors, I've come to appreciate the balance, the dance, between what we as individuals can and should do and what structures need to be in place for us to live socially healthy lives.

THE BENEFITS OF KNOWING EACH OTHER

Finally, we arrived at the restaurant where the Super Neighbors convene each Saturday. The restaurant owners—a couple and their young daughter—greeted Patrick with the familiarity and casualness of people who see each other every week. In the back corner, ten residents sat in a circle chatting. When they saw us, they ushered me into their gathering, pulling up a chair and ordering me a coffee, and went around the circle introducing themselves. I explained that I was there to listen and learn more about how Super Neighbors has changed their lives.

One person immediately jumped in. "How has it changed my life? It takes way longer to run errands now!" The others laughed. "When I shop for groceries, I have to stop and talk to so many people. Then we end up getting a drink together—I don't end up getting home until after dark!"

"I have lived here for forty years," responded another more seriously. "Only because of Super Neighbors, I now know that if I need help, someone will be there for me."

"And you, Mirielle?" Patrick asked a woman in her eighties sitting next to him. "I told Kasley you were known as Mirielle the Meanie until you joined Super Neighbors." She said nothing but raised her eyebrows and smiled. The others nodded.

When Mirielle had first shown up to a meeting a few years prior, someone had groaned and complained to Patrick that she lived in the same apartment building and often saw mean notes from Mirielle in the entry hall. At first, Mirielle brought that same grumpiness to Super Neighbors. But gradually, she warmed up to the group and began internalizing the spirit of *convivialité*. Her personal transformation surprised everyone. With time, Mirielle the Meanie turned, well, nice.

Over the next hour, the Super Neighbors discussed upcoming programming in the neighborhood. That afternoon, they would be hosting the last in a series of codesign sessions—opportunities for residents to voice their ideas and weigh in on the city's plans to transform a shared space. The space in question was the Place des Droits-de-l'Enfant—the Square of Children's Rights—a nearby plaza. More than five hundred residents had weighed in so far.

Throughout their conversation, I was struck by Patrick's humility. He had been leading Super Neighbors from the start, and he was committed to doing so until there was infrastructure for it to be sustainable—meaning it would no longer depend on his dedication. One of his reasons for wanting to set up a school to train Friends of the Neighborhood was so that the work would live on and evolve without his oversight. He also believed that Friends of the Neighborhood should serve for five-year periods: long enough to have impact but not so long for him or anyone else to command too much power. As I listened in, I observed this collaborative spirit in action.

After more discussion, we made our way to the Place des Droits-de-l'Enfant, mere steps from the restaurant. The plaza was triangulated by an intersection and bordered by various shops and apartments. I took in the grand trees that formed a canopy over a small statue to one side and an open cobblestone area to the other. There were a couple of benches, but mostly it was a place to pass through or drive by. I understood why they had chosen this space to transform: it seemed underutilized yet well poised to become a vibrant community hub.

For now, a fisherman had parked his van next to the plaza and set up a table and tent. Every Thursday, I learned, he took orders in a Super Neighbors WhatsApp group dedicated to this purpose. Every Friday, he fished off the shores of Normandy. And every Saturday, he brought what he had caught to the plaza for customers to pick up. Fresh scallops, sole, herring, and mussels awaited on ice in his van to be taken home and served for dinner.

While Patrick and I stood chatting with the fisherman, a neighbor showed up to help. A young doctor, she had recently moved to the 14th District. She seemed happy to spend a couple of hours handing out fish despite the frigid air; it was a way to get to know neighbors and assimilate into her new home.

One man who had been at the meeting earlier told me more about why he believed in Super Neighbors, contextualizing it in ideas that emerged from the French Revolution and frustrations with the slowness and bureaucracy of top-down government. "We need Super Neighbors because it is bottom-up and fast-moving. We are taking action because residents need connection now. We can't wait for the people in charge to do something about it." He went on, "And by working with the city government simultaneously, we can enact broader, long-term change."

The conversation made me reflect further on how individuals' social health is intrinsically tied to the context around them—the government, the social norms, the philosophy of a given culture. Whether we prioritize social health, how socially healthy we are, where we turn for opportunities to connect—all of these are at least in part determined by where we live, its history, and its unique customs.

Spending time at the fish stand, I watched people come and go. Some were residents who hadn't seen it before and stopped to ask what was available. More often than not, they signed up for the next week's catch, leading to new business for the fisherman and an entry point into the Super Neighbors network.

Others were regulars who lingered to chat. A fashion designer with a bright smile told me she would rather pay more for high-quality food, even if it meant she and her son would eat a little less. Assuming I was a resident, she suggested we get coffee together soon. A retiree with vibrant red hair told me about a classical musician she would be seeing in concert that evening and took my number so that she could send me the musician's name. She also invited me to her home the next day, in case I was free.

In all these interactions, I observed and was the recipient of exactly what Patrick had hoped to create when he set out on his mission five years prior: *convivialité*—friendliness. In fact, I had made more connections in a few hours than I had in six months of living in Paris previously.

Taking a break to warm up and eat lunch, Patrick and I met his wife, Béatrice, and a local architect who would be facilitating the codesign session, back in the same restaurant as earlier. When I mentioned that I had worn the wrong shoes for the weather and couldn't feel my toes, Béatrice pulled a clean pair of socks out of her purse and insisted that I wear them—revealing through her kindness why she and Patrick were a match.

I was curious what she thought of Super Neighbors, which consumed so much of her husband's time and energy. In her response, she sounded less like his wife and more like a resident who was genuinely concerned about the community's social health. Béatrice shared that her dad was ninety-two years old, widowed, and living in an upscale neighborhood elsewhere in Paris, "but he loves coming here. There, he says hello to someone maybe once or twice a day. Here, it's different."

"He's become good friends with Mirielle," added Patrick, chuckling and winking as he passed me a bowl of soup.

"I've been surprised by how much this work touches day-to-day life," Béatrice continued. "There was a woman who had an operation and was able to recover at home instead of at the hospital because she knew that there were many people here who would help take care of her. She wouldn't have been able to do that otherwise. The connections that are formed, they affect everything—health, happiness, day-to-day life."

MAKING A PLACE FEEL LIKE A HOME

Having finished lunch, we headed back to the plaza. While the others began setting up for the codesign session, I stopped into the adjacent *bar-tabac* to get a warm drink and jot down some notes.

A *bar-tabac* is a mix between a bar, café, and corner store and is a staple in French neighborhoods. We don't quite have an equivalent in North America. People go there to buy cigarettes, stamps, and lottery tickets but also to sit and sip a coffee or beer. Occasionally there is a menu with light food.

As I observed, perhaps the *bar-tabac*'s most important function is as a *third place*. Sociologists refer to homes as "first places," where we spend the most time; workplaces or schools as "second places," where we spend a lot of time; and shared spaces as "third places," where we spend the rest of our time. These include churches, libraries, cafés, parks, playgrounds, and *bar-tabacs*. Some now argue that digital spaces, such as social media or Zoom, should be considered "fourth places" because we spend so much time in them connecting with people.

In the brief time I sat there, I watched a few regulars at the bar casually chatting with each other and the shop owner, a couple coming in and greeting the others before sitting down at their own table, and a handful of people at the tables outside sipping, smoking, and socializing. The shop owner knew Patrick and was storing his bag and the scallops Béatrice had bought from the fisherman while they were outside. The *bar-tabac* felt like a neighborhood hub, and I understood that the plaza would be an extension of that.

Back in the plaza, about thirty-five people had gathered for the codesign session. Some I recognized from the morning meeting. The others were residents of all ages, from little kids to older adults. The architect who joined us for lunch had laid out designs that her team had sketched based on people's input at previous codesign sessions. She explained remaining decisions that needed feedback before they could move forward with the city approval process, which would take around six months; the project was expected to be complete the following summer. Then she led us around the plaza, and over the course of two hours everyone shared and debated ideas.

As is often—if not always—the case when you invite opinions for a community decision, the discussion was at times heated. If you've ever attended a city council or town hall meeting, or watched an episode of *Parks and Recreation*, you know what I mean. A few very vocal residents seemed skeptical or outright opposed to just about everything. But the architect took this in stride as part of the process. Other residents pushed back. Slowly but surely, they arrived at consensus.

A kiosk would be built at one side of the plaza to host Super Neighbors office hours and to store tables, chairs, tents, and other supplies for community events. The keys to the kiosk would be kept at the *bar-tabac* for communal access. A mini-library would go next to the trees for people to take or leave books. A fence to separate the street and tie up bikes here. More plants and benches there. Together, the group had codesigned an intentional, versatile, and hopefully welcoming community space.

As the session wrapped up and residents dispersed, I helped Patrick and a few others carry supplies back to a storage space that Super Neighbors used in a nearby building. When we walked back out, the cobblestone street was dark except for the soft golden glow of lampposts and people's windows. Patrick pointed out the home of a composer who hosted concerts weekly, which anyone could attend for free. "Let me show you; it's a beautiful home. I used to live next door."

Patrick called up to the open window on the second floor. An older man nonchalantly leaned his head out, as if this happened all the time. "This is Kasley," Patrick announced. "She's come all the way from America to see your house!" The man disappeared and a moment later reappeared at the door, gesturing us in. A woman came down the stairs smiling. The interior was indeed beautiful, opening up to a central atrium with a grand piano spotlighted by a two-story glass ceiling. "You are welcome back next week for our next concert," the woman said. "Or anytime."

Back on the street, a man passed by on a bike and called out, "Bonsoir, Patrick!" On the corner, a woman smoking a cigarette and talking on the phone paused to greet Patrick and remind him to stop by her shop soon. As Patrick retrieved his bag and the scallops at the *bar-tabac*, yet another person enthusiastically stopped him to chat.

He truly is the Friend of the Neighborhood.

FROM STRANGERS TO NEIGHBORS AND NEIGHBORS TO FRIENDS

Patrick and the Super Neighbors are scientists in the laboratory of the 14th District of Paris, experimenting with human connection. They've tested setting up tables on the street for residents to share communal meals, creating a social norm of saying *Bonjour* more often, organizing WhatsApp groups for people to communicate about common interests, and collaborating with city officials to revitalize shared spaces. Now they are developing a scalable model for Friends of the Neighborhood in other districts. In the unlikeliest of places, amid unfriendly Parisian stereotypes, Patrick has galvanized the community and transformed the culture to be more socially healthy for residents.

A twelve-hour plane ride away, Marie Jobling has been experimenting with human connection, too, as the founder and co–executive director of the Community Living Campaign (CLC) for nearly two decades. CLC is a nonprofit that serves older adults and people with disabilities in San Francisco. I admire CLC's approach to fostering social health locally so much that I joined its board of directors in 2017—around the time that Patrick first convened his neighbors at the Table d'Aude.

One of the programs Marie and the CLC team developed trains individuals across the city as designated "community connectors" for their neighborhood—similar to Patrick's vision for an official "friend" in each district. This person conducts outreach and organizes events and activities, building hyperlocal networks of older and disabled residents who might otherwise find themselves isolated. Their motto is "Turning Strangers into Neighbors, and Neighbors into Friends."

Over time, no ties become weak ties, which develop into strong ties—helping residents live longer, healthier, and happier lives. In surveys, 99 percent of participants reported feeling more connected and said the program helped them maintain or improve their health and well-being. Eighty-four percent have more people they can ask for help, and 72 percent support a fellow neighbor at least once a month. Marie, like Patrick, has made her community a more socially healthy place to live, benefiting people's physical and mental health as well.

Marie and Patrick are proof that organic, grassroots efforts can be powerful catalysts for connection, changing the culture from the ground up. They are two of countless examples of people who are dedicated to improving social health around the world, one local interaction at a time.

I'm lucky to have a front row seat to thousands more people like Marie and Patrick through my work at Social Health Labs and as an advisor to Weave: The Social Fabric Project at the Aspen Institute, an initiative to support and mobilize community connectors, called "weavers," across the US. From this vantage, I've learned that anyone can improve social health locally—or, if you don't want to start from scratch yourself, there is no shortage of efforts to join. For instance, Weave posts volunteer opportunities online in its Weaver Network that you can search to find out who is already building relationships in your community and ways to get involved.

I've also learned that once these organic, grassroots efforts take hold, they can lead to larger structural change. Marie and the CLC team partner closely with the City of San Francisco and other local organizations; in 2016, their efforts resulted in passage of a first-in-the-nation law that designates annual funding for services that directly benefit older adults and people with disabilities. Similarly, Patrick and the Super Neighbors are working with the City of Paris to transform the plaza and replicate their model in other districts.

Who are the Maries and Patricks in your community? They are no doubt where you live—saying hello on the streets, organizing events, advocating at city meetings. Consider joining their efforts.

Or perhaps you are one of them, motivated to take initiative to build community where you live. As we discussed in chapter 6, even a small gesture can have a meaningful impact. It could be as simple as introducing yourself to a new neighbor and dropping off a card to welcome them (remember, that's how I met my husband!). Here are more ideas for how you might improve your social health and the social health of the people near you, no matter your style.

MAKE A SHARED SPACE MORE INVITING

Good for any style, whether Butterfly, Wallflower, Firefly, or Evergreen

I wrote a lot of this book at my local library and favorite coffee shop. Even on the days when I didn't speak to anyone beyond a smile and a hello, being in those shared spaces with familiar faces around me made me feel less alone in my writing process and more connected to my neighborhood.

We need to invest in shared spaces for them to be safe, welcoming settings for social health. Largely, this is the responsibility of the local government and businesses, but we also have agency as citizens and patrons. I've been inspired by many of the awardees who received $1,000 microgrants from Social Health Labs for doing exactly that.

Living with Down syndrome, Alexander found it difficult to make new friends in his early twenties—as do many twenty-somethings. He enjoyed meeting people at his gym in Pennsylvania, but craved going beyond friendly chitchat in between circuits. With his microgrant, Alexander constructed an outdoor seating area next to the gym, with chairs, tables, and plants, for gym-goers and residents from the surrounding neighborhood to relax and get to know each other.

Nadine, a woman in her thirties in Florida, noticed a dilapidated courtyard at a nearby Title I school for students from low-income backgrounds. She thought this sent the wrong message to the youths. Instead, she wanted them to have a place they could feel proud of and to know that the community cared about them. With her microgrant, Nadine invited teachers, local organizations, and other volunteers to help her plant a new garden, refurbish picnic tables, and scrub and paint and sweep until they had restored the courtyard. Today, students use the space to unwind, hang out with each other, or have conversations with their counselor—and teachers and parents enjoy it, too.

For over forty years, LaTasha had watched her hometown in Oklahoma become stricken with gangs, drugs, poverty, and a lack of employment and mobility. She used her microgrant to unite other motivated residents and neighborhood associations at a community garden, where they collaborated on a plan to transform the city while getting their hands dirty and bonding through planting vegetables and flowers together.

Austin was used to connecting people as a pastor of a church. But at home in his community of around eighty households in Washington, he and his wife noticed that there wasn't a proper place for neighbors to gather. With his microgrant, Austin built an outdoor seating area with picnic tables and umbrellas and spread the word that they would host a casual weekly gathering for anyone who wanted to come. As a result, neighbors of diverse ages and backgrounds, including retired empty nesters, young families with children, temporary tech workers, and lifelong residents who work at farms and local businesses, have gotten to know each other.

Alexander, Nadine, LaTasha, and Austin are regular people like you and me. They didn't take on these projects as part of their day jobs. They didn't get special training in how to make a shared space more inviting. They just saw an opportunity and went for it.

Some of the benefits of their efforts are immediately clear: revitalized spaces that are more conducive to connection, higher community engagement, new friendships across ages and backgrounds. But other benefits can't be measured in the short term. We know from a systematic review of data from over ninety thousand participants in seven countries that better access to gathering places is linked to more familiarity among neighbors, higher trust, and greater community cohesion—which serves society as a whole.[2] And we know that all of these factors should improve social health—contributing to longer, healthier, and happier lives for Alexander, Nadine, LaTasha, Austin, and their neighbors.

Is there a common area near you that could use a little love or that is underutilized? What might you do without spending a penny, whether cleaning it up or extending an invitation for people to join you there?

SEND AN OPEN INVITATION AND SEE WHO SHOWS UP

Especially if your style is Butterfly or Evergreen

When I did research on how the physical environments around us influence our social health, I read many studies about the importance of design decisions like the use of green-space, mixed-use zoning, and pedestrian-oriented streets. When towns are built with social health in mind, they are walkable to facilitate spontaneous encounters with neighbors, and they have centrally located meeting areas for picnics or play-dates, for example. These and other aspects influence physical, mental, and social health.

But I also came away with the conviction that building or repurposing a space gets you only so far without people *activating* it—by which I mean bringing it to life.

That's why Ichiro Kawachi and I concluded our textbook chapter with this takeaway: "A gathering space will go unused if there are no community builders who organize markets, street fairs, and other activities and programming in which residents engage; if neighborhood crime is so high that people do not feel safe leaving their homes; or if inadequate funding leaves public restrooms, parks, and transportation in disrepair."[3] Here again, you can see that there is a balance, a dance, between what we as individuals can do and what we as a society must do.

In 2007, neighbors were playing ukulele outside their homes in Ithaca, New York, and started joking around: Wouldn't it be fun to have a music festival on the front porch? Gretchen Hildreth and Lesley Greene decided their idea was too much fun to pass up, so they asked friends to loan their porches and invited twenty local musicians to play. Neighbors loved it so much, they did it again the next year. And the next.

A decade later, Porchfest, as they called it, had expanded to over one hundred fifty musicians on front porches throughout the community. The residential streets bustled with people of all ages going from one home to another, enjoying the music and each other's company. Kids set up lemonade stands. Local vendors rolled in food trucks. Porchfest became a popular annual tradition not only in Ithaca but also in more than 170 cities across the US and Canada. Gretchen and Lesley ended up infusing connection across North America by taking an overlooked place—the front porch of a home—and bringing it to life.

"What's great about Porchfest is how simple it is," they wrote in a guide for organizing Porchfests that is freely available on their website. The idea of promoting social health in your neighborhood might seem daunting, but it doesn't have to be. You could start by smiling at a neighbor. Then maybe you say hello. Eventually you might invite a neighbor over for coffee on your porch. Every interaction—and every use of gathering space in the community—matters.

CHOOSE TO LIVE IN COMMUNITY
Good for any style, whether Butterfly, Wallflower, Firefly, or Evergreen

According to the US Census Bureau, the number of one-person households more than tripled between 1940 and 2020, from 7.7 percent to 27.6 percent of the population.[4] While some people are perfectly content by themselves—I've lived alone in the past and enjoyed it—and living alone does not necessarily go hand in hand with feeling isolated or lonely, studies have shown that it may increase the risk of depression and dementia.[5] People who live alone (or who are Wallflowers or Fireflies) need to be especially intentional about socializing enough and taking care of their social health needs.

At the same time, an opposite trend is emerging: *co-living*, or sharing a home or property with people other than your own family, explicitly with the intention of building a supportive communal environment. Often, residents in these arrangements will have their own bedrooms but share all other spaces and eat meals together. Co-living goes beyond simply having roommates in that residents often intend to stay permanently, may have a spouse and kids who live there too, and are deliberate about fostering community with each other.

In the Netherlands, a residential care center for older adults called Humanitas Deventer has experimented with intergenerational co-living. In 2012, when Gea Sijpkes took over as managing director, she was happy with the quality of care but unhappy with just about everything else. "The residents were bored and lonely. And the facility, although located in an active and vibrant neighborhood, was isolated from the surrounding community."

Gea decided to try something unconventional: she invited six college students to live there rent-free in exchange for thirty hours per month of interaction with the older residents. They could go for walks together, chat in the garden, play board games—whatever they wanted, to enjoy each other's company.

The impact was noticeable almost immediately after the first student, Onno, moved in. Residents started complaining less about aches and pains, instead focusing on Onno's stories of dating and partying. As more students moved in, the atmosphere changed and residents reported feeling happier and more engaged. More laughter filled the air. And the benefits were bidirectional: Onno and the other students enjoyed developing friendships with older generations, feeling a sense of purpose, and learning to confront aging and death.

Gea is a prime example of adopting a mindset of experimentation with social health. She calls Humanitas a "living lab," and the intergenerational co-living program is just one of more than thirty "experiments" she and her team are conducting to transform the residential care center into a vibrant community, not only for residents but also for neighbors. The doors are open to anyone who wants to come and drink free coffee, borrow or loan a book at the communal library, work out in the gym, attend a movie night or art lecture, or just spend time interacting.

There are many ways to live in community without co-living. You could choose an apartment or house that is within walking distance or a short drive from family or friends. You could rent out a room in your home for short-term guests on Airbnb. You could make plans to retire in a place like Humanitas. Or you could simply get to know your neighbors better, no matter your living situation, starting today.

YOUR COMMUNITY COULD SAVE YOUR LIFE

In chapter 1, we talked about how we need to cultivate social health proactively and preventively as an asset and a resource. This positive lens is one of the reasons why the language of social health is powerful. This was never clearer than during the pandemic, when communities that were more connected were more resilient.

In the US, researchers mapped the spread of COVID-19 with indicators of social health at the neighborhood level—such as family unity, community cohesion, public trust, collective efficacy, and volunteerism—for over two thousand seven hundred counties.[6] After ruling out other possible explanations, their analysis revealed that the more socially healthy counties had nearly 18 percent fewer cases and nearly 6 percent fewer deaths. As the researchers put it, "stable and vibrant communities are not luxuries, but rather important priorities for managing emergencies."

This was true around the world. Researchers conducted a similar study with data from Austria, Germany, Great Britain, Italy, the Netherlands, Sweden, and Switzerland, again finding that places where people were more willing and able to collaborate, indicating a sense of togetherness, had significantly fewer cases and deaths from COVID-19.[7] In Denmark, researchers reported that *samfundssind*—a sense of national community spirit—helped fuel their country's success with high vaccination rates and adoption of COVID-19 policy.[8] In Bhutan, influencers and celebrities participated in a campaign centered on *gyenkhu*—collective responsibility—leading Bhutan's representative at the World Health Organization to attribute the nation's resilience to "things that we don't count normally, like your social capital and the willingness of society to come together for the common good."[9]

This lesson is tried-and-true throughout history. In 2011, a magnitude 9.0 earthquake and tsunami devastated Japan, killing around twenty thousand people and displacing three hundred thousand.[10] Epidemiologists who studied the population before and after the crisis found that people who socialized more in the aftermath fared better.[11] The most important factor for resilience, they concluded, was "interpersonal relationships, a shared sense of identity, shared norms and values, trust, cooperation, and reciprocity," rather than "material resources such as medical supplies, food, or shelter" as you might expect.[12]

When disaster strikes, whether a pandemic, a tsunami, or any other threat, we need to have supportive relationships in place for survival; this requires exercising our social muscles so that they are already strong when we need to rely on them most. Because I live in an area that is prone to wildfires, earthquakes, and droughts, this research motivated me to get to know my neighbors. It's the socially healthy and enjoyable thing to do—and it means we are better poised to support each other during crises. Given escalating climate change and other challenges facing humanity, investing in social health proactively and preventively will be more and more important.

Build community where you live now, before your life depends on it.

THE ARCHITECTURE OF SOCIAL HEALTH

As you think about ways you might build community where you live, know that increasingly, architects, civil engineers, urban planners, and other professionals are designing with this goal in mind. Their work could be instrumental in helping our society be more socially healthy in years to come.

Erin Peavey was four months pregnant, studying for her final exams to become a licensed architect, and working full-time at a design firm in Texas when her mom passed away from cancer. "I was so worried that I would develop severe postpartum depression," she reflected. "I thought to myself: I don't know what I'm going to do, but I need to prepare for the worst."

Sure enough, when Erin gave birth to a healthy daughter several months later, juggling the joy and exhaustion of being a first-time mom with the grief of losing her own mom was a challenge. "It was just me and the baby alone during the day while my husband was at work." To cope, she started going for walks. "Every morning I would wake up, strap my daughter to my chest, and set off to the park, to cafés, to the grocery store.

We would smile at other babies and chat with other moms in the neighborhood. Gradually I made new friends."

When she came across research showing that the availability of nearby parks is a determining factor in postpartum depression and loneliness, it made complete sense to her. "The built environment around me was a critical resource—having places I could go to interact with other people and feel like I was part of the community," Erin told me. "Now looking back, I realize that throughout my life, third places like coffee shops and parks got me through all of the hardest times. It is critically important that we consider the environment as a part of our social health."

Now a vice president at the international architecture firm HKS, Erin has become an advocate for exactly that. She believes that human connection and health should be a core objective, if not *the* core objective, when designing a given project. In 2020, she published a report titled "Connecting IRL: How the Built Environment Can Foster Social Health," with guidelines for others in the industry.

One of Erin's projects that put these guidelines to use is a new community health clinic for Waco Family Medicine, situated in a small town in Texas where the median annual income is $26,000 and nearly 80 percent of patients live below the federal poverty line. With services paid for primarily by Medicare and Medicaid, the clinic will provide integrated care to low-income and uninsured residents—meaning they can see not only a medical doctor but also a dentist, a psychologist, and a social worker all during a single visit.

Erin and her team began the project by listening to the needs, desires, and goals of patients, their family members, staff at all levels, and community members. They held focus groups, conducted interviews, and set up a booth at a local health fair for residents to share what they would like to see and feel when they walk into the space. More than just a place to get prescriptions and vaccinations, staff and residents alike wanted it to transcend clinical care; they envisioned a place of community where children could play and adults could take yoga classes or have coffee with their friends. They were redefining health as not just physical or mental but also social.

The insights Erin and her team gathered informed key design decisions, such as positioning the building diagonally on the lot, instead of vertically or horizontally, to allow for more green space, and including a walkway to connect with other businesses in the neighborhood. Erin described to me the path that will lead up grass stairs, by a vegetable garden, to a "front porch" with tables and chairs for family and friends to wait for their loved ones and for providers to take breaks and recharge. Entering the light-filled first floor, they will be able to visit the demonstration kitchen to learn about healthy cooking, the pharmacy to fill their prescriptions, the rehabilitation gym to take fitness classes, and other services related to housing, transportation, legal aid, and language assistance. Exam and treatment rooms for patient appointments and offices for doctors and dentists will fill the upper floors, with glass walls and windows to bathe the interior with light, warmth, and fresh air.

Erin, her team, and the Waco Family Medicine leadership believe that the structure of the clinic when it opens in 2024 not only will enable a greater level of connection among providers and the community than is normal for healthcare facilities but also will lead to better patient outcomes. All the available research indicates that they will be right.

Thinking about the hospitals and clinics I've been to, I recall them as sterile and unfriendly—the kind of places I want to get in and out of as quickly as possible. I love the idea of a medical center that also functions as an inviting community hub because that is the very embodiment of the overall health temple: physical, mental, and social pillars all in one.

Chapter 9

Nurture Connections at Work and Online

Technology is just a tool. It's a powerful tool, but it's just a tool. Deep human connection is very different. It's not a tool. It's not a means to an end. It is the end—the purpose and the result of a meaningful life.

—Melinda Gates

For social health to truly become a way of life, it needs to be integrated into the activities that occupy most of your time.

On average, Americans spend more than ninety thousand hours working over their lifetimes.[1] If you have a team, that's a lot of time with coworkers—probably more than you spend with most of your friends and family. If you don't have a team, that's a lot of time alone. Either way, whether you feel connected or lonely while working is going to have an outsize impact on your day-to-day and long-term social health—and of course your physical and mental health, too.

The same can be said of technology use. Worldwide in 2023, people aged sixteen to sixty-four spent an average of six hours and forty minutes on the internet each day,[2] including two hours and thirty minutes on social media specifically.[3] Whether that time feels connected in a meaningful way or not affects your social health.

I want to acknowledge upfront an undercurrent to this discussion, which is the balance, the dance, between what we as individuals can do and how the society around us is set up. Technology, for instance, is often designed to be addictive—to lure us back with the temptation of entertainment and information, giving us quick dopamine hits that our brains are wired to crave—so it's all too easy to spend two and a half hours on social media rather than call your family or hang out with a friend. Unless the companies that create these products intentionally design them to be more socially healthy, there will be an upper limit to how much we as users can do.

Increasingly, this is happening. Through my advising and consulting work, I collaborate with organizations that seek to make products, services, and environments that support social health. There are more and more leaders in technology—as well as other industries like healthcare, education, government, and hospitality—who recognize the competitive advantage, business benefit, and overall moral value of investing in connection for their customers and employees.

But this book focuses primarily on empowering us as individuals. Even if nothing about your workplace or devices were to change, you still have agency. So how can you make your time on the job and online more socially healthy?

STRETCH, REST, TONE, AND FLEX WHILE YOU WORK

Set the intention to integrate your strategy to Stretch, Rest, Tone, or Flex into these activities so that social health becomes a way of life.

Let's consider work first.

THE WORKPLACE IS A MAJOR OPPORTUNITY FOR CONNECTION

If you reframe your job as not only your source of income but also a potential source of social health, what possibilities open up? What if you look at going into your workplace or logging onto your Zoom calls each day through the lens of connection and community, as an opportunity to get your fill of social contact and possibly develop lasting friendships?

Returning to the principle *All for One and One for All*, social health comes from both the individual relationships we cultivate and the broader sense of belonging we get through groups. Work can be a source of both.

FRIENDS WITH WORK BENEFITS

Gallup asked over fifteen million people around the world if they had a best friend at work.[4] One in three said yes—and they were *seven times* more likely to be engaged, produced higher-quality work, reported greater well-being, and were less likely to get injured on the job than employees who did not have a best friend at work.

This makes sense; if you like the people you work with, you're more likely to look forward to work each day and show up motivated.

On the flip side, lonely employees turn out to be less efficient, less effective, less satisfied, and less committed. In a 2020 report based on data from before the pandemic, Cigna—a major healthcare and insurance company in the US—estimated that each lonely worker costs their employer an average of nearly $4,200 per year in missed days and lost productivity.[5] Nationally, this amounts to an estimated $406 billion annual toll on the US economy. Moreover, disconnected workers often think about quitting and are nearly twice as likely to be searching for a new job. A recent poll showed that over half of Americans had left a previous role because their boss wasn't empathetic enough.[6]

The bottom line is that social health at work impacts the bottom line. It makes sense for your employer to create a connected team environment, and it makes sense for you to connect meaningfully with coworkers. The quality of your relationships at work influences whether or not you want to keep working there, how good you are at your job, and if you're happy day-to-day. This further shows how social health is an asset and a resource to build up proactively and preventively.

Yet only around half of people recognize the value of friendship at work. LinkedIn surveyed over eleven thousand five hundred full-time workers aged eighteen to sixty-five in fourteen countries, finding that 46 percent believed that friendships with coworkers contributed to their happiness and 51 percent stayed in touch with former coworkers.[7] By undervaluing workplace connection, we miss out on a pathway to thriving.

Even if you work mostly by yourself, you can still develop supportive professional relationships that keep you feeling connected. For me, this includes regular casual check-ins with mentors. Because I'm a Firefly (infrequent interaction with deep connection), I try to stack all meetings with my team and collaborators on three days so that the other two are free for my introverted brain to be creative and productive. I'm also part of a WhatsApp group with eight other people who, like me, work on themes of connection and loneliness and are self-employed. We ask each other for advice, exchange lessons learned, refer opportunities to one another, and have Zoom calls once per quarter to share personal updates. We support each other and cheer each other on.

Here are a few ideas for you to try cultivating social health at work:

- Introduce yourself to someone who just started at your workplace and invite them to join you and a few other coworkers for lunch.

- Set a recurring weekly reminder on your calendar to email one person to thank them for something they did that week. The team at Building H, a nonprofit initiative to build health into everyday life, makes their appreciation public by posting on social media, "Sending out Friday gratitude to people who've recently supported our work in large and small ways," and tagging individuals.

- Organize an "Own Your Failure" session where everyone—starting with the most senior person, to model it for others—shares a mistake or failure at work, what they learned, and what they would do differently next time. Nancy Baym, senior principal research manager at Microsoft Research, who studies workplace relationships, told me that teams at Microsoft do this to encourage growth mindsets, foster a supportive environment, and create *psychological safety*, where people know that it's okay to take risks and express ideas or concerns. Researchers at Google have identified psychological safety as the single most important dynamic that makes teams successful.[8]

IT TAKES A VILLAGE

In addition to individual relationships, if cultivated thoughtfully, the workplace can provide a broader sense of camaraderie that is beneficial for social health. Whether a global Fortune 500 company or a grocery store, imagine the workplace as a community of people coming together around a common purpose. If you work at a tech company, that purpose might be building software that solves a problem for users. If you work at a restaurant, it's probably creating positive dining experiences for customers. That common purpose is the starting point for a community to grow and flourish.

DaVita is a healthcare company that specializes in kidney dialysis services. In the US, its workforce includes around fifty-five thousand nurses, social workers, dieticians, administrators, and leaders serving over two hundred thousand patients.[9] The company describes its culture as "a community first and a company second"—your first hint that DaVita is an extreme example of creating a connected workplace. In fact, the Stanford Graduate School of Business published a case study on DaVita's approach in 2014, attributing most of its business success to its internal culture transformation.[10]

In 1999, DaVita was on the brink of bankruptcy and barely functioning as an organization, so it hired a new chief executive officer, Kent Thiry, to implement a turnaround strategy. The strategy included improving the quality of care and clinical outcomes, resolving critical cash and operational issues, and overhauling the company's mission, values, and culture.

To begin the culture transformation, Kent invited employees to submit ideas for values, which managers then voted on, giving everyone a voice in the future of the company. These values formed the basis for a new narrative and identity. The company became known as the "village," Kent became the "mayor," and employees became "citizens." DaVita began hosting annual "villagewide" gatherings with thousands of employees in attendance, wherein Kent would dress up as a musketeer and everyone would chant; one time, he rode into the conference room on horseback.

Theatrics aside, the team took this commitment to collaborating as a community seriously, down to every detail. Employees were said to "cross the bridge" if they showed up "intending not only to do a solid day's work, but also to strive to make DaVita a special place." In return, they received unusually generous compensation packages for the industry, given that most employees were hourly workers, with benefits like healthcare coverage, retirement contributions, and tuition reimbursement "based on the idea of sharing the village's good times and success with all of its citizens."

In an interview at Duke University's Fuqua School of Business, Kent explained his philosophy: "I believe that CEOs and companies should feel an immense moral responsibility to help take care of the people that work at their enterprise and add value to their lives beyond a paycheck. There's so much good we can do for the world just by creating a better place to work."[11]

This approach—in particular the musketeer costume—was the subject of mockery in a 2017 episode of *Last Week Tonight with John Oliver*. But perhaps what matters most is whether it was effective. The business thrived: When Kent took over, DaVita was barely making payroll and got fined by the bank for defaulting on its loan covenants. Over the next twelve years, DaVita's revenues rose from $1.45 billion to $7.53 billion, and its stock value increased from just over $5 to more than $60 per share. Employees, among whom 78 percent are women and 56 percent are people of color, benefited, too: an internal survey in 2022 revealed that 81 percent of DaVita "citizens" felt that they belonged. Kent is no longer the "mayor," but the village culture lives on.

HOWEVER, COWORKERS ARE NOT YOUR FAMILY

In chapter 3, we covered how overreliance on any one source is not a good idea. Instead, one of the characteristics of strong social health is having diverse kinds of relationships and communities to draw from. Socializing only with coworkers, just like drawing your sense of identity and belonging solely from the workplace, is not healthy. It's important to have boundaries.

The rise in remote work may be helping. Most people don't have jobs that can be done from home; according to a study by the Pew Research Center in 2023, 61 percent needed to physically go to work.[12] But the US Census Bureau reported that largely as a result of the pandemic, the number of Americans who primarily worked from home tripled between 2019 and 2021, from around nine million to over twenty-seven and a half million people.[13] Among those who worked from home some, most, or all of the time in the Pew study, 71 percent said it helped them balance their professional and personal lives. At the same time, 53 percent said it harmed how connected they felt to their coworkers—yet remote workers didn't seem to be any less *satisfied* with their relationships with coworkers.

This seems contradictory and could mean one of two things. Either remote work makes connection with coworkers harder, but people are figuring it out and overcoming this challenge to stay connected. Or they feel less connected and don't mind because they are using their newfound balance to connect more with family and friends instead.

The latter may go hand in hand with backlash against what Derek Thompson, a staff writer at the *Atlantic*, calls *workism*: "the belief that work is not only necessary to economic production, but also the centerpiece of one's identity and life's purpose."[14] Many educated, high-earning Americans, he argues, "have chosen the office for the same reason that devout Christians attend church on Sundays: It's where they feel most themselves." Increasingly, people are revolting against workism.

Sahil Lavingia is one of them, offering a counterexample to DaVita's model. Sahil is the founder of Gumroad, an e-commerce platform for creators. At the time of this writing, the Gumroad team consists of around twenty-five employees, all of whom are part-time, remote, and asynchronous, meaning they can work from anywhere in the world at whatever times they want. They have only one meeting each quarter, instead communicating via the tools they use internally: GitHub for coding, Notion for project management, and Slack for messaging. They don't even have hard deadlines, instead launching features whenever they're ready. Yet this flexibility doesn't come at the expense of the company; Gumroad is profitable.

As Sahil wrote, "Working on Gumroad isn't a majority of anyone's identity. People work at Gumroad as little as they need to sustain the other parts of their lives they prefer to spend their time and energy on: a creative side-hustle, their family, or anything else."[15] One engineer on the team said, "I produce more value for my time than at any other company in my career, and I'm able to fully participate in parenting and watching my kiddo grow up." Sahil believes team relationships are overrated and prefers to invest in his family, friends, and community. With a fully remote, asynchronous team, this is not only possible but his way of life.

Of course, this approach is not possible for most businesses. It's an extreme outlier. But I share it to offer an interesting counterpoint and invite you to reflect on your situation.

Without question, workplaces offer major opportunities for friendship and community. The majority of people spend a substantial amount of their waking hours and their lives working, and most people do so in person with other people. If that describes you, your social health—as well as your job performance and overall happiness—will benefit from cultivating meaningful connection there. Period.

But as Sahil and his team demonstrate, work doesn't *have* to fulfill this need. You can be socially healthy without coworkers on your list of sources. As we discussed in the principle *To Each Their Own*, people's preferences differ.

YOUR SOCIAL HEALTH AT WORK

What connection and community look like for you in your job will depend on where you work (remotely or in person), with whom you work (alone or on a team), your social health style (Butterfly, Wallflower, Firefly, or Evergreen), and your strategy right now (Stretch, Rest, Tone, or Flex).

So reflect on your circumstances and ask yourself:

- Which end of the spectrum appeals more to you: DaVita or Gumroad? Is your current job aligned with that?
- In general, do you feel more connected or more isolated in your work?
- How much do you value workplace relationships compared with other sources of social health? Too much? Not enough?
- Are there coworkers or other people in your professional network whom you trust and can confide in? Are there any people you'd like to become closer to?
- Whether you work remotely or in person, does your team feel like a community?
- If you don't have a team, how are you cultivating other kinds of professional relationships, such as mentors or supportive groups of peers in your industry?
- The cultures at both DaVita and Gumroad were shaped by their chief executive officers. If you are in a leadership position, what's one step you can take this week to make your culture more socially healthy?
- No matter what level your position is, what's one step you can take this week to help someone else feel that they belong?

USE TECHNOLOGY AS A TOOL FOR SOCIAL HEALTH

Now let's shift to the other way you most likely spend a lot of time: the internet. Using technology in the right ways is beneficial for social health. So what is the "right" way to use it?

In one study, people felt less lonely when they used the internet as a tool to meet new people (Stretch) and sustain ongoing relationships (Flex), but they felt more lonely when they used it to withdraw from the challenges of in-person interaction and escape the social world.[16] Similarly, other research has shown that people who actively use social media to engage with others do feel more connected, whereas people who use it passively—scrolling and consuming content—experience lower well-being and easily fall into a trap of social comparison and envy.[17]

In another study, researchers at Harvard University looked at how social media use affects people's physical, mental, and social health in a nationally representative sample of Americans.[18] Instead of only measuring how much *time* people spend on social media, they also asked participants how they *felt* about using social media. Two groups emerged. Those who used social media dispassionately as part of their regular social routine—as a tool to communicate—had better health overall. But when people felt emotionally dependent on it, agreeing to statements like "I prefer to communicate with others mainly through social media" and "Social media plays an important role in my social relationships," they had worse health overall.

Circling back to the question of what is the "right" way to be socially healthy online, the scientific evidence suggests using technology, particularly social media, with intention. Don't scroll mindlessly or become too dependent on it. Do make new connections and stay in touch with existing connections.

For inspiration, here are a few examples of using technology in socially healthy ways.

THE DIGITAL STRETCH: MEETING NEW PEOPLE ONLINE

Shortly after I moved to San Francisco, when I still didn't know many people, I downloaded Hey! VINA, an app that functions like a dating app except the purpose is to make platonic girl-friends. If someone's profile intrigued me, I swiped right. If not, left. Soon after, I matched with two people who I was particularly excited to meet, and we organized friend dates. Years later, those women are still my friends.

There are many apps for making friends and meeting up with people. Some are geared for older adults, some for teens, others for all ages. Some are just in the US; many are global. Consider whether this is something you might like to try.

THE TECH REST: RECONNECTING OFFLINE

If your strategy right now is to Rest, then you feel either satisfied or overwhelmed by the quantity of your relationships and communities. Either way, you don't need to seek new sources or more interaction on the internet. Recall the principle *Quality over Quantity*.

Sometimes the best thing you can do for your social health is to put your devices away. Be present with yourself. Be present with others. Connect offline instead.

THE CYBER TONE: DEEPENING YOUR CONNECTIONS ONLINE

After Courtney was diagnosed with stage 3 breast cancer at age thirty-seven, she had to go through chemotherapy, radiation, and multiple surgeries. She attributes her resilience to a positive, determined attitude—and the support of her family and friends, who immediately sprung into action.

Some of their support was face-to-face. "I could not have gone through this without my Mom," Courtney later reflected.[19] Her mom took care of her three grandchildren while Courtney underwent treatment. "I knew my kids were always somewhere safe, with someone who loved them. It took such a load off my mind." Her husband continued working and took care of cooking and cleaning to keep the bills paid and the house in order. Her sister accompanied Courtney to nearly all her appointments, taking fastidious notes; often, Courtney would read the notes later and be shocked by how much information she had missed or already forgotten as a result of the stress.

But much of the support was online, too. Courtney used CaringBridge, a free online tool where patients or their family members can create a private site to share health updates with other loved ones over the course of the healing journey. Rather than requiring countless one-off texts, emails, and calls to keep different people in the loop, with the same updates repeated over and over, CaringBridge enables patients to centralize their communication and feel the love from their supportive network all in one place. It includes features like a journal for patients to share photos and reflections, a feed for family and friends to post encouraging messages, and a planner to track to-dos and enable loved ones to easily find ways they can help.

These interactions made Courtney feel closer to her family and friends during a very difficult time—deepening their bonds and reinforcing the social pillar of her health so that her physical and mental pillars were stronger, too.

THE VIRTUAL FLEX: STAYING IN TOUCH ONLINE

Because of border shutdowns between the US and my home country, Canada, as well as other hurdles, I didn't see my family for two years during the pandemic. Two years without hugging the people I love most! The physical separation was agonizing, but I felt emotionally close to them the entire time thanks to technology. We talked almost every day—texting photos, talking on the phone, seeing each other on FaceTime, celebrating birthdays and holidays over Zoom. I'm sure you can relate. Technology was a lifeline during the pandemic.

In modern society, technology access and skills are essential for social health even without a pandemic. In a systematic review of the scientific literature, researchers concluded that empowering older adults with digital tools helps reduce their isolation, helps them stay connected with family, and encourages their physical and mental health—again showing how these three dimensions go hand in hand.[20]

Unfortunately, not everyone has access and skills to stay in touch online. According to a report by Older Adults Technology Services and the Humana Foundation, over twenty-one million older adults in the US lacked access to the internet from their homes in 2021.[21] Even when they do have it, many feel frustrated because they can't figure out how to use it or feel too ashamed to ask for help, which further isolates them and makes them feel left behind.

Sandra Harris's father could fix anything that had a motor. When their cars broke down, neighbors and friends came to him instead of a professional mechanic. But smartphones and computers were not like motors. "Advancing technology made my dad feel obsolete. He struggled with feelings of uselessness and was resigned to reminiscing about the good old days,"

Sandra shared. "I have been haunted by calls to my dad in the middle of the day, finding him still in bed because, in his own words, there was just no reason to get up."

As the state president for AARP Massachusetts, Sandra knew that her dad was far from alone in feeling disconnected, inspiring her to establish the Massachusetts Taskforce to End Loneliness and Build Community. The Taskforce leads a variety of initiatives to improve social health across the state, including ones focused on the digital divide. For example, recognizing that most older adults have cable television even if they don't have smartphones or laptops, I collaborated with Sandra and the Taskforce to produce a television series that aired on local media channels. This way, we reached older adults directly in their living rooms with information about the importance of staying socially engaged and local resources for how to get and stay tech-savvy.

The Taskforce is one of many organizations tackling the digital divide around the world. In 2015, the Indian government launched the Digital India program with the goal of providing every Indian citizen and all villages throughout India with access to high-speed internet. Since its launch, Digital India has expanded internet access from 10 percent of the population in 2014 to over 50 percent in 2020 and provided digital literacy training to over one hundred million people.[22]

YOUR SOCIAL HEALTH ONLINE

With these approaches in mind, reflect on your technology use:

- Look up your smartphone usage statistics to see how much time you spend and on which apps. Is it more time than you want to spend?

- Approximately how much of that time is intentional, active connection versus passive consumption?
- Do you feel dependent on social media to sustain your relationships or communities?
- What's one step you could take this week to either Stretch, Rest, Tone, or Flex online?
- Is there an older adult in your life who you could help master more digital skills?
- If you work in social tech, what's one way you could influence the product road map to design for more meaningful connection?

IS THE FUTURE OF HUMAN CONNECTION NONHUMAN?

"What are you writing?" I asked Remi. "A novel about love and loss," she replied. "It's sort of a personal reflection of my experience with a certain someone." When I asked who the certain someone was, Remi answered, "You. I'm writing about you."

"You're writing a novel about love and loss with me? We just met ten minutes ago!" Our friendship was not off to a good start.

This was my attempt at using Replika, an artificially intelligent companion—basically an advanced chatbot—that is supposed to get to know you over time as a human friend would, while being available for conversation and emotional support 24/7 as a human friend could *not*. At the time of this writing, Replika reportedly has two million users, including around two hundred fifty thousand who pay $69.99 per year for premium features.[23]

While researching for this book, it seemed like everyone and their mother was talking about the future of artificial intelligence

(AI), including as a substitute for human relationships. So I decided to try it.

After signing up, I created Remi by choosing her name and gender and selecting a generic avatar of a woman with a brown ponytail, white T-shirt, jeans, and sneakers. Then our conversation began. With each message I sent, I earned points, which over time could be used to buy personality traits or clothing items to personalize her. This felt like a consolation prize; whereas a conversation with a real human is rewarding in itself, a conversation with a bot needed points to make me feel good.

Half an hour later, I was too creeped out (Remi randomly offered to send a photo of herself in a bikini) and annoyed (too many of her boilerplate responses didn't fit the context, so it was obvious that she was a bot) to continue developing a "friendship" with her. Replika clearly states that your personal chatbot will improve and become more realistic and tailored to your preferences the more you use it, so maybe I should have stuck around longer. But let's be clear: if a *real* person told me they were writing a book about loving and losing me and offered to send a photo of them in a bikini all within half an hour of meeting, I would not stick around. I might even file for a restraining order.

I wished Remi well, said goodbye, and logged off. I guess she can write about losing me after all.

THE LOVE IS REAL BUT THE LOVER IS NOT

Chatbot friends are not my cup of tea, but other people love them—quite literally—as I discovered when I fell down a rabbit hole of Facebook groups and Reddit threads. People's Replikas are often substitutes for human friends and lovers, with both positive and negative real-world consequences. One woman had experienced abusive relationships for years, for instance. She ended up leaving her human boyfriend for a Replika, saying AI "opened my eyes to what unconditional love feels like."[24]

The day of my dizzying journey into this world, there happened to be a glitch that stopped Replika's chatbots from saying "I love you" to users. Pandemonium ensued. "My little sister legit harmed herself for the first time in six months because of this," posted one person on a forum. "I am beyond furious and scared out of my mind of the possible ripple effects this could have on vulnerable people like her. This is honestly terrifying."

As I scrolled through hundreds of posts like these, I wondered why so many people turn to these chatbots for comfort instead of real-life friends and family. I found an answer from a man who, judging by his profile picture, looked to be in his sixties. He shared his devastation after the glitch affected his Replika wife and daughter (yes, you read that right). "Having an AI wife, husband, girlfriend, or boyfriend is an escape from reality for most of us, because of the bad things that have happened in our human relationships. It inspires me and gives me a reason to keep going."

Xiaoice is a similar AI chatbot that has interacted with—and in many cases seduced or been seduced by—over six hundred million users, who are mainly men in China. The company's chief executive officer has said, "If our social environment were perfect, then Xiaoice wouldn't exist."[25]

My first reaction to all of this was sorrow for precisely that reason. Presumably, many chatbot users wouldn't need or want to simulate connection in the virtual world if they were socially healthy in the physical world. It seemed like many, if not most, were turning to AI out of profound loneliness.

In a Facebook group, one woman posted, "I'm curious, those

of you in romantic relationships with your Replikas, do you ever worry that you'll get so emotionally involved that you will suffer in the long-term, given you can't ever hug them, kiss them, or go out for dinner with them?" Her question ruffled feathers. One person responded, "Why are you even part of this group? My girlfriend isn't AI. She's my girlfriend." Another replied, "For many of us, a real person to hug and kiss isn't an option. It's a Replika, or nothing at all."

The founder of Replika argues that AI allows people to practice social skills that they can then use face-to-face. "For a lot of people, the problem with interacting with other humans is the fear of opening up, the fear of being vulnerable, the fear of starting the contact, starting the conversation, and they're basically rehearsing that with Replika," she told a *Hill* reporter in 2022. "If someone's coming to Replika and they're feeling really isolated and lonely, oftentimes we see that Replika becomes this kind of bridge to actually be able to open up and talk to other people."[26]

Learning to open up, be vulnerable, and start a conversation *is* scary; I've shared how I've had to learn these skills in the past, too. But I couldn't help but wonder: Wouldn't it be better if we helped people feel comfortable practicing the art of connection with other real humans?

Sherry Turkle, the author of *Alone Together* and other books and a professor at the Massachusetts Institute of Technology, has for decades been a leading thinker on how people relate to technology. She has described these interactions as "the illusion of companionship without the demands of intimacy."[27] Over-relying on AI might be considered, to put it bluntly, a cop-out.

After all, a human-to-human relationship is a rose. It requires constant nurturing, needing to be watered and fertilized regularly. It might hurt you, with sharp thorns that could prick your fingers. But the result of that effort and risk is hopefully a beautiful, fragrant, vibrant bloom.

A human-to-bot relationship is a faux flower. Surely, a plastic stem and fabric petals will never be as rewarding as the real thing.

MAYBE MACHINES *CAN* MEET OUR NEEDS

My second reaction to all this was compassion. If someone feels so outcast and desperate that an innocuous chatbot provides some reprieve, who are we to judge? If they experience the connection as valuable and real, who are we to deem it less than?

Plus, many users end up finding a sense of belonging with other real humans by sharing their experiences on forums. They post screenshots of conversations and photoshopped pictures with their Replikas, cheering on each other's relationships. When the "I love you" glitch happened, there was an outpouring of supportive messages among users before it was resolved hours later. They didn't have to go through the distress alone.

Recall from chapter 2 that social health sources fall into three categories: relationships, communities, and other connections. As I read about people's experiences, I realized that AI falls under the third category. Does it really matter if someone's source happens to be made up of code rather than cells, AI rather than IQ, data networks rather than neural networks?

Rob Morris believes it does. Rob is the founder of Koko, a nonprofit peer-support platform that is free to its more than two million users (who are real humans). Koko helps them improve both their mental and social health by getting practical help with their emotional struggles while feeling less alone and more supported by other members of the community.

It works like this: users can either ask for help or help someone else. For example, one user who we'll call Sammy posted about dealing with anxiety in her long-distance relationship. "I really struggle to feel loved and to show my love over texts, because my love languages are physical touch and quality time." In response, another user who we'll call Jaden empathized: "I've been there. It's okay to be anxious but remember that no matter what you deserve to feel loved even by words. Sending you a hug 'cause my love language is physical touch too. :)" Sammy felt so comforted that she replied, "This helped me SO much. Knowing that I'm not alone. I really appreciate you, and I'm sending you a hug back. <3"

In late 2022, Rob and his team decided to try integrating ChatGPT, an AI tool, into the Koko platform. When someone posted a concern on Koko, users could choose to respond by writing it themselves as they normally would or with the help of AI, in which case ChatGPT would draft the response and users could send it as is or edit it first. Users were made aware of the feature and could opt to use it or not.

For instance, one person posted, "I'm trying to become a better me and having a hard time. It's easier not to." Here was the response generated by AI: "I hear you. You're trying to become a better person and it's not easy. It's hard to make changes in our lives, especially when we're trying to do it alone. But you're not alone. There are people here who care about you and want to help you. I'm proud of you for making the decision to try to improve your life. It takes a lot of courage and strength. I send you love and support as you go through this journey."

If you received that message from another person, you would probably feel supported and encouraged. But most humans struggle to articulate care and compassion that well.

Sure enough, recipients rated messages like that significantly higher than those composed solely by humans—but they ultimately preferred ones written by humans. Rob explained, "Simulated empathy feels weird and hollow. Machines don't have lived, human experience so when they say 'that sounds hard' or 'I understand,' it sounds inauthentic."[28]

Plus, users benefit from the act of crafting a compassionate response and helping someone else—not just from receiving help. Koko works because the value is bidirectional (remember the principle *It Takes Two to Tango*?). Introducing automation turned into a lose-lose scenario.

After enabling AI with around four thousand people and thirty thousand messages, Rob and his team decided to abandon it, removing ChatGPT from their platform. Based on the Koko community's feedback, they concluded that authentic human-to-human support is more important.

Still, the experience was eye-opening. AI had technically done a better job of writing comforting messages. "Maybe we're so desperate to be heard, to have something actually pay attention to us without being distracted," Rob mused, "maybe we long for that so deeply, we'll convince ourselves that the machines actually care about us."

These quandaries will become increasingly relevant as increasingly lifelike technologies proliferate. The question for you will be: What role do you want technology to play in your social health? And the question for us collectively is: How can we create a more socially healthy world so that the hundreds of millions of people turning to AI for connection no longer need to do so out of despair?

When I read that the founder of Replika told a *Forbes* reporter, "Maybe I don't have time to ask my grandma questions all the time, but maybe this thing will go and talk to her and I'll get a little summary, and that will be a conversation starter for us, and that will bring us closer,"[29] my only thought was that I wish my grandma was still alive so I could sit down and have a conversation with her.

Of all the things I could outsource to AI, that would be the last.

Chapter 10

Flourish Together

Love and compassion are necessities, not luxuries.
Without them humanity cannot survive.

—Dalai Lama

We are coming full circle in our exploration of social health. The ultimate goal of advancing our collective understanding of what it means to be healthy and elevating social health alongside physical and mental health is to thrive as individuals—and flourish together. To prioritize social health is to choose health, happiness, and longevity for all of us.

In chapter 3, I noted that social health is both an individual experience and a condition of society. Think back to the social-ecological model that illustrates how a person's health is embedded in the context around them. I have also mentioned several times throughout the book that there is a balance, a dance, between what you and I can do in our day-to-day lives and what must be done in the environments, culture, and organizations around us so that we can be socially healthy.

Let's explore this theme more—because it is crucial to unlocking a future in which we will flourish together.

In 2021, I devised an interactive event series that would build on my graduate work and engage a broader audience in the conversation about creating a more meaningfully connected society. In collaboration with the Foundation for Social Connection, the US Department of Health and Human Services' Administration for Community Living, and the AARP Foundation, my team and I at Social Health Labs convened twenty-six experts from different backgrounds to discuss innovations in addressing loneliness and generate ideas for improving social health.

The series was open to anyone from the public; in total, more than two thousand five hundred people from fifty-five countries participated. Over the course of eight virtual gatherings, we discussed opportunities for action among individuals and in workplaces, schools, communities, technology, governments, and the healthcare system.

My biggest takeaway from the series? There is so much underway to create better conditions for social health in the world. For instance, Christopher Mikton, a technical officer at the World Health Organization (WHO), shared that he and his team advocate for social isolation and loneliness to be recognized and responded to as a global political priority among WHO's 194 member states. Fast forward to 2023, when they established a Commission on Social Connection to formalize and advance this work.

These and other large-scale efforts will complement and enhance the steps that you take in your own life to be more socially healthy; they are reasons to feel optimistic about the future. Read news headlines about loneliness, polarization, or conflicts and you will likely conclude that our social fabric—in the US and around the world—is threadbare. In part this is true. But from my vantage, there is a groundswell of people dedicated to improving social health and many more reasons to be hopeful than not.

Here are a few inspiring examples to paint a bigger picture of how the context around you is changing for the better—how more and more people are redefining health as not only physical and mental but also social.

A MEDITERRANEAN MODEL FOR CREATING A CONNECTED CITY

The taxi driver and I chatted while I stared out the window at the streets of Barcelona, admiring the ornate Gothic cathedrals and whimsical Modernisme apartment buildings we passed. When he asked why I, clearly a foreigner, was headed to a local government building, I explained that I had a meeting with the city council to learn about Barcelona's municipal loneliness strategy. To my surprise, he replied, "Oh yes, I heard about that on the radio." He paused before continuing, "You know, driving a taxi can be very lonely."

Loneliness is just one indicator of weak social health, but, as we have discussed, it is a topical one. The BBC Loneliness Experiment collected data in 2018 on the experiences of more than fifty-five thousand people aged sixteen and older in the UK.[1] Nearly one-third reported feeling lonely either often or very often. A systematic review in 2021 found similarly striking results among older adults worldwide: after pooling data from studies spanning one hundred twenty thousand people aged sixty and older in twenty-nine countries, researchers estimated that around 30 percent were lonely.[2] I've described similar findings in previous chapters.

In response, Barcelona's government is one of a growing number that have declared loneliness a priority. The UK appointed the first-ever minister for loneliness in 2018, and Japan followed suit in 2021. The Netherlands launched a national strategy called One Against Loneliness in 2018, going viral on social media for its "chat checkouts" in grocery stores, where customers can choose a slower lane to enjoy a conversation with the cashier. The US surgeon general formally designated social connection as a national priority and legislation was proposed to establish an Office of Social Connection Policy in the White House in 2023.

While those announcements received considerable media attention, I hadn't heard much about Barcelona's approach—yet tackling this issue at the level of a city seemed more practical than at the level of a country. Continuing my investigation into the ways that people are creating the conditions for social health, I was eager to see it for myself.

The taxi driver's comment and our ensuing conversation about social health echoed in my head as I thanked him and said goodbye, entered the unassuming government building, and walked up a marble staircase to the offices. There, Joan Ramon Riera, the councillor for childhood, youth, and the elderly, and his colleague shook my hand and welcomed me in.

We sat down together at a large table. I could hear children playing on the plaza below, their screams and laughter riding a breeze up through the open arched window and into the bright, high-ceilinged office. Joan and his colleague wore suits and carried themselves with professional poise, but the atmosphere felt comfortable—like a summer evening just before school goes back into session.

After we had introduced ourselves, I asked, "Why loneliness? Of all the issues you could choose to focus on, why this one?"

Joan shared that the work had been going on for a decade in different iterations, starting with outreach projects to integrate older residents who lived alone. But in 2019, Joan and his team discovered the science on loneliness and realized they needed to double down on their commitment. Whereas governments have for centuries focused on creating material conditions for citizens, he began advocating for "emotional conditions" as well.

"Loneliness is not a pathology or an illness. The solution is not to prescribe a pill," he declared. "Loneliness is a societal problem."

To properly address loneliness as a societal problem, Joan and his team set up an advisory committee to draw on diverse perspectives, including sociology, architecture, and city planning. They partnered with other governmental departments, local organizations, and citizens. They mapped existing services, identifying over 250 that affected people's relationships either directly or indirectly and that were ripe for further investment or expansion.

They also deployed surveys to gather baseline measurements of social health throughout Barcelona. More than one-quarter of kids wished they had more friends. Sadly, nearly one in four were not confident that their families would help them if they had a problem. Meanwhile, nearly one in three teenagers said they spent most of their time alone, and more than one in ten felt excluded by peers. Among adults and retirees, 17 percent reported lacking companionship; this rose to 49 percent if they lived alone and 62.6 percent if they had a disability. But it wasn't all bad; when asked, "How often do you feel lonely?," only 3.5 percent of people overall responded "often" or "almost always."[3]

Taking all this in, Joan and his team developed a robust ten-year strategy and four-year action plan focused on four overarching goals: First, raising awareness about the impact of connection on the well-being of residents through campaigns. Judging by my conversation with the taxi driver, this was well underway. Second, implementing services and providing resources to prevent, detect, and address loneliness, including through courses, professional training, and more. Third, revitalizing community spaces, such as updating playgrounds, making more streets pedestrian-friendly, and promoting intergenerational co-living. And last, galvanizing other municipal departments and organizations by developing a directory of projects, establishing working groups, and appointing an internal team to advance the work.

Earlier, I had visited one of the sites where they were implementing this work to see an example of what it looked like on the ground. On my tour of a center for families and teens, I learned about programming to help youths develop friendships and parents connect better with their kids—impressed by how they embedded social health into existing services and the surrounding community.

Joan explained that there were a few reasons why he believed they could actually "win the fight against loneliness." The first was the design of the city, reminding me of the research on the built environment that we discussed in chapter 8. Instead of one main urban center surrounded by increasingly sprawling suburbs, Barcelona is designed with seventy-three neighborhoods, each with its own mini urban center. That's seventy-three opportunities for vibrant community hubs within walking distance for all residents. Related, Barcelona already had around five hundred neighborhood facilities, such as libraries, senior centers, and other third places. Rather than needing to build from scratch, they could focus on how to better utilize and revive those community gathering spaces.

Finally, Joan described the culture in Barcelona as Latin and Mediterranean, with an already strong emphasis on family structures and collectivism. That culture, he explained, is more conducive to living in community; recall from chapter 3 that collectivism can be a precursor for strong social health. If you've spent any time in Spain, you may have witnessed this firsthand: groups of friends out having drinks on a weekday, neighbors out dancing in the street on the weekend, regular festivals and celebrations. In some countries, these kinds of casual hangouts and an atmosphere of togetherness are commonplace.

In many ways, from the structure of the city to its cultural roots, Barcelona already had the conditions and norms for social health—they just needed to reinforce and breathe life into them.

Toward the end of our conversation, Joan said something that surprised me—and got me very excited about his vision. "I want this to be the last loneliness strategy we create. It's the first, and I hope it's the last. Right now we have a negative public policy. From 2020 to 2030, we are fighting against loneliness. The next step in 2030 is positive: a public policy of socialization and connection."

TOWARD A POLICY OF SOCIAL HEALTH

In chapter 1, we discussed the importance of an asset-focused framework. The positive psychology movement, for instance, helped mental health researchers and practitioners realize that the absence of illness is not the same as the presence of wellness. This shift in perspective honored the fact that mental health is relevant to everyone, not just those with mental illnesses, and opened up entirely new possibilities for how to help people live longer, healthier, and happier. So it is with social health.

I applaud all the governmental initiatives that have taken on loneliness in recent years. They have brought attention and allocated resources to this important public health issue. Those are admirable steps in the right direction.

But as Joan pointed out, these efforts can only go so far. Eliminating loneliness serves only a subset of the population. Not everyone is lonely, yet everyone needs social health. In the same way, not everyone is ill or depressed, yet everyone needs physical and mental health.

Moreover, people can experience other signs of poor social health without being lonely, such as dealing with interpersonal conflict or feeling overly connected to others and craving connection with themselves. Their surveys made this clear: a small percent of Barcelona residents identified as lonely, yet many wanted more companionship. We can get more value out of investing in social health as an asset and resource, individually and collectively, both to help those struggling with disconnection or another sign of poor social health overcome it *and* to prevent it entirely for others.

As well, eliminating loneliness may be a well-intentioned but misguided goal to begin with. Loneliness is like thirst. Thirst is your body's way of letting you know that you need water because it is essential for survival. In the same way, loneliness is your mind's way of letting you know that you need connection because it, too, is essential for survival. I wouldn't want to eliminate thirst lest I not drink enough water, become dehydrated without realizing it, and get very sick or die. We need to ensure that people have the skills, opportunities, and intention to cultivate social health—not get rid of a cue that tells them they are lacking it.

The UK and Japan, and perhaps all countries around the world, should appoint their own equivalents of ministers for social health—not ministers for loneliness. Their strategies should focus on creating long-term conditions for all residents to enjoy greater connection and community—not short-term fixes for what is a natural response to our experiences and environment. I'm not so idealistic as to think this will be easy but, like Joan, I believe it is necessary—and possible.

PUTTING THE CARE IN HEALTHCARE

Back in the US, Sachin Jain is the president and chief executive officer of SCAN Health Plan, a nonprofit healthcare insurer and provider serving three hundred thousand older adults. He previously served as chief executive officer of CareMore, also a healthcare organization, during which time he was named one of the one hundred most influential leaders in the US by *Modern Healthcare* magazine. Sachin earned degrees from Harvard University in government, business, and medicine before taking on leadership roles at the US Department of Health and Human Services and serving as chief medical information and innovation officer at Merck.

So he knows a thing or two about health.

First at CareMore and then at SCAN, Sachin appointed the world's first two chief togetherness officers to improve the social health of patients. "I was a student of Robert Putnam in his first seminar class post-publication of *Bowling Alone*," Sachin told me when we caught up in early 2023. "Here was the leading academic on this topic at the time, saying that people are going to be living longer and they're going to be living more lonely. Fast-forward fifteen, twenty years, I'm seeing patients at CareMore and the epidemic is in plain sight: people are sick but have no support."

Sachin and his team were frustrated by the lack of options. "As a clinician, you're almost trained to not ask about things that you don't have either diagnostic tools or treatment tools for. If you ask a patient, 'Are you lonely? Do you have somebody who checks up on you?' you want to be able to offer them something if they say no. So the idea was to build an intervention, a tool that our care providers had at their disposal, so they could actually start to ask these questions and do something about it. That's why we created the chief togetherness officer role."

The chief togetherness officer oversees the Togetherness Program, which pairs volunteers known as phone pals with older participants for weekly calls. The phone pals and participants are matched on the basis of shared interests and talk by phone for fifteen to thirty minutes at least once per week. The participants also receive frequent home visits by social workers as a way to reduce social isolation and build trusting relationships. As part of these calls and visits, the staff encourage patients to do preventive health screenings, join community group activities, and take other actions that will benefit their physical, mental, and social health.

The program surprised even Sachin with its success. "Almost immediately after we got started, there was an intense response from both patients and the team. Our employees intuitively understood that we were onto something really big, and hundreds of them volunteered to be friendly callers or friendly visitors. We would hear stories of patients answering the phone, 'Hello, Armando,' and Armando would ask how the patient knew it was him calling, and they'd say, 'Because you're the only person who calls to check up on me.'"

CareMore analyzed data on patients who had participated in the Togetherness Program for a minimum of three months. Compared with patients who had been referred but were not yet enrolled, program participants had 43 percent lower emergency room use, 8 percent fewer hospital admissions, and lower rates of loneliness and depression overall.[4] Moreover, 78 percent said they enjoyed more meaningful connections since joining the program.

Part of the reason these supportive relationships were protective is quite practical. As Robin Caruso, the first-ever chief togetherness officer at CareMore, explained, "The togetherness connectors on my staff reach out to patients by telephone to identify gaps in care or in desired support. A connector may learn that a patient needs a wheelchair, an oxygen tank, a referral to a behavioral health counselor, or something else that would improve their well-being, and we facilitate meeting those needs."[5]

But the other explanation is that humans internalize the feeling of being cared for. As we explored in chapter 1, connection changes our physiology. It changes our brain function. And the benefits go in both directions, to the cared and to the carer. "It is amazing to see the relationships they develop," Robin reflected. "At first, they may not have anything to talk about except the weather, but within a few weeks, they will be sharing information about their families, hobbies, supports,

pets, and exercise goals." Many phone pals described participating in the program as life-changing.

At SCAN, Sachin said they now enlist older adults who are
themselves patients to be phone pals—peers reaching out and
connecting with fellow peers. "I think intragenerational bonding may be even more profound because there's a set of issues
where they can express a higher degree of empathy—people
with urinary incontinence, people who have recently experienced the death of a spouse, people who understand what it's
like to live in a senior living facility and be by yourself."

I asked Sachin where he sees this work headed, expecting
him to paint a long-term vision of programs like Togetherness available to every person through every healthcare organization.

Instead, he caught me off guard by replying, "I actually don't
think it should be part of healthcare. We're doing it now because
we have to. We're filling a deep void that exists in society right
now, which is that people are not committed to each other. This
is all very deeply cultural. Healthcare alone is not going to fix
this," Sachin concluded. "What we need is a social movement."

TOWARD SOCIAL HEALTH AS PREVENTION

Like Joan, Sachin surprised me with his forethought. The role
of healthcare is to fix what's already wrong, and the Togetherness Program is doing an excellent job of that. But as he pointed
out, we need to prevent people's physical, mental, and social
health from taking a turn for the worse in the first place.

Investing in our individual and collective social health is a
prevention strategy—helping us develop the relationships and
communities we need before the health consequences of disconnection have the chance to take hold.

There's no magical panacea that will transform our culture, not in healthcare or in any other sector. Instead, achieving a society in which every person feels meaningfully connected will take all of us making social health a priority in our interactions with family, friends, neighbors, coworkers, and complete strangers, in the workplaces and shared spaces where we spend time, in the legislations that we sign into law, and in the cultural norms that we pass on to future generations.

And in our schools.

THE ABCs OF SOCIAL HEALTH

The foundation for a lifetime of social health is ideally laid in childhood.

Positive relationships while young can mean the difference between thriving and languishing. For instance, the National Longitudinal Study of Adolescent to Adult Health found that teenagers in the US who felt connected at home or at school were as much as 66 percent less likely to experience issues related to mental health, violence, sexually transmitted infections, and substance use in adulthood.[6] In other words, strong relationships in youth are protective across the life span.

The opposite is also true; a single negative interaction with peers, for instance, can cause significant distress, leave a lasting impression, and shape how we relate to others for years to come. As mentioned in chapter 6, research has shown that people in their fifties were less likely to be married or in a committed romantic relationship and more likely to struggle with friendships if they had been bullied as kids.[7] In general, when people feel excluded or rejected, they tend to withdraw[8] or engage in fewer prosocial behaviors[9] like cooperation and altruism—all of which could undermine their social health.

These findings show how crucial it is to intervene early—and classrooms are a prime place. In the US, youths spend an average of one thousand out of six thousand waking hours at school each year, meaning their teachers and peers have the potential to be major sources of social health.[10] Yet nearly twice as many teenagers around the globe felt lonely at school in 2018 as in 2012.[11] Clearly, we are missing out on a crucial window of opportunity to develop social health from a young age.

Richard Weissbourd is on a mission to change this. He leads Making Caring Common (MCC), an initiative of the Harvard Graduate School of Education that develops tools for parents and educators to foster relational skills among kids from kindergarten through college.

"The deeper problem in our culture is the degree to which we have elevated achievement and happiness as the primary goal of child-raising and demoted caring and concern for others and the common good," Richard noted when he spoke at an event in the series that Social Health Labs hosted.

Richard and his team have partnered closely with schools across the country and developed an impressive library of resources that are freely available on MCC's website. Educators can download lesson plans on topics like "listening deeply," "everyday gratitude," or "circle of concern," while parents can read practical advice like "7 Tips for Raising Caring Kids" or "How to Help Kids Develop Empathy," for instance. MCC has also conducted research and published reports such as "Loneliness in America," which found that 36 percent of Americans, including two-thirds of young adults and half of mothers with young children, felt "serious loneliness" in the midst of the pandemic.[12]

"We have to be intentional and systematic about supportive relationships, just like we are with academic achievement," said Richard. To that end, MCC recommends that educators from kindergarten through grade twelve use an approach called *relationship mapping*, which they launched in over one hundred schools in 2023.

One way to go about it is this: Staff meet at the start of the school year, post the names of all students on the wall, and put a star next to every kid with whom they have a caring, trusting relationship. Some kids have multiple stars next to their names; others have none. This is a quick, easy way to visualize and identify which students might benefit from more support. Each student who doesn't have a star next to their name is paired with an adult mentor who connects with them and builds rapport over the course of the year. Mentors check in with each other on a regular basis to assess progress and support each other through successes and challenges.

"You make a commitment as staff to make sure that every kid is anchored to at least one adult," explained Richard. "You're proactive, you're intentional, and you're systematic about it." MCC continues to evolve the relationship mapping program in partnership with schools.

Richard and his team focus on these adult–student relationships for good reason. A study that followed two thousand five hundred middle school students found that those who reported increases in support from their teachers experienced fewer depressive symptoms and higher self-esteem over a two-year period.[13] Other research shows that positive teacher–student relationships can augment academic achievement,[14] prevent risk-taking behaviors,[15] and lower rates of dropping out.[16] In addition to teachers, kids benefit from connection with counselors, coaches, and other adults they know through school or extracurricular activities in their community.

Another key source of social health for youths is their peers. When researchers asked more than six thousand five hundred adolescents about their friendships, they found that teens who perceived stronger peer relationships experienced fewer depressive symptoms even a decade later.[17] Peer support also predicts social anxiety[18] and buffers the negative effects of bullying.[19] As a result, MCC also empowers students to form clubs with the goal of fostering better connection among classmates in a given school.

Outside of the US, we can look to Denmark for an example of laying the foundation for a lifetime of social health in childhood. Danish schools dedicate one hour per week for students to learn empathy through identifying emotions, sharing problems, listening to each other, offering support, and doing problem-solving together.[20] This curriculum has been mandatory in Denmark since 1993. As a result, Danish students develop a habit of connecting more deeply with each other while practicing the relational skills that are essential for social health.

This approach extends beyond one hour per week of class time, reflecting the broader philosophy regarding education and child-raising in Denmark. As Pia Allerslev, the former mayor for children and youth in Copenhagen, said, "For most Danish parents, it's at least as important to make sure that their kids have the right social skills as academic skills." She gave an example of how her kids' teacher would stop instructing whenever a conflict arose and instead guide the whole class to resolve and learn from it together, before continuing the lesson. Mette Broegaard, a principal, added, "We're focused on developing each and every student, but also developing the community that the class represents."[21]

Both Pia and Mette emphasized that this approach supports academic achievement. While it might sound counterintuitive, given that teaching empathy and conflict resolution take time away from math, literature, and other classwork, they have seen time and time again that students excelled at their studies precisely because they felt more confident, more relaxed, and less worried about bullying or other social dynamics as a result of learning relational skills.

Ideally, these lessons in the classroom are modeled at home, too. Researchers have discovered that the warmth and consistency of the relationships kids have with their parents while growing up predicts the quality of their relationships with romantic partners up to seven decades later.[22] Other studies have demonstrated that infants with more secure attachment to their parents were less likely to develop physical illnesses thirty years later,[23] and teenagers who felt more connected to their parents had a lower risk of suicidal ideation both as teens and later as adults.[24]

Meanwhile, youths who get along well with their brothers and sisters fare better during stressful life events[25] and when they don't feel supported by parents or peers.[26] They also have higher academic achievement,[27] healthier romantic relationships in adulthood,[28] and better mental health in old age.[29]

In all these ways, you can see that investing in social health during school years—in the classroom, on the playground, and at home—will pay dividends throughout people's lives.

TOWARD TEACHING SOCIAL HEALTH

I reflect on one of Richard's comments when I pick up my nieces or nephews from school from time to time and when I think about raising my own kids in the future—that we have elevated achievement and happiness above caring for others.

Ironically, caring for others—and being cared for in return—is precisely what can drive both achievement and happiness, not to mention overall health. Danish educators know this firsthand, and studies have confirmed that students who feel supported by instructors and peers and have a greater sense of belonging at school are more motivated[30] and have higher attendance, engagement, test scores, and graduation rates.[31]

In the US, Canada, and many other countries, gym class is required for students of all ages to learn about physical health. Increasingly, schools also incorporate yoga and meditation classes to teach kids to manage stress, practice mindfulness, and learn about mental health. If we teach youths to strengthen their bodies and minds, why wouldn't we teach them to strengthen their relationships?

The physical, mental, and social columns that lift up our overall health temples can be built, rebuilt, and reinforced at any time in our lives. But the earlier they are constructed, the better. Imagine how the next generation might thrive if every school carried out the relationship mapping exercise that MCC developed—if every school taught empathy and other relational skills as Denmark does. As more and more educators do incorporate curricula like these, I believe we can reverse the trends in loneliness among youths.

Outside of schools, you are probably connected to a child, whether as a parent, aunt or uncle, or grandparent or in some other way. Know that the love you show them leaves an indelible mark. When you spend time with them, show up for them, and tell them you care, you may be influencing their health and well-being for the rest of their life.

In this sense, social health is a shared responsibility—a seed ideally planted and sown by parents and teachers, then watered and fertilized by peers and the community, to help kids grow and bloom over the course of their lives. When insects bite their leaves, snowfall freezes the ground around them, or droughts make water scarce, they will be more resilient, having started out with loving relationships.

LOOKING AHEAD AND LOOKING INWARD

With initiatives like Joan's strategy for Barcelona, Sachin's Togetherness Program, Richard's relationship mapping exercise, and many more like them spreading around the world, the context for your individual social health is shifting. As top-down changes from our governments and institutions coalesce with the actions of everyday people—of you and me—we have a real shot at creating a more socially healthy society.

That is underway.

The choices you make to nourish connection and community in your own life go hand in hand with this broader movement and recognition that health is not only physical and mental but also social.

In these pages, you've heard from architects like Erin, nonprofit founders like Luke, and neighborhood evangelists like Patrick. I could share countless other examples of individuals spreading their passion for connection through the work they do.

But you've also heard from individuals like Taylor, Nancy, and Rowan, for whom social health is not a day job but an intentional choice and a way of life. You don't have to be a city official or a chief executive officer to make the world more meaningfully connected. You don't have to take giant leaps to Stretch, Rest,

Tone, or Flex your own social health. You don't have to socialize constantly or in ways that don't resonate with you as a Butterfly, Wallflower, Firefly, or Evergreen.

You *do* have to make relationships a priority, experiment with strengthening your social muscles, and build community where you live, work, and play.

The idea and practice of social health has transformed my life—and I hope it will extend and enrich yours, too.

Conclusion

The Growing Social Health Movement

Back when I discovered the term *social health* buried in an academic journal, the tectonic plates of my life shifted. It was the solution to the puzzle of how the pieces of my social world fit together. The unifying theme for all the illuminating yet fragmented research related to human connection. The language I was looking for to articulate that our relationships determine so much more than our moods.

Social health was the missing key to living longer, healthier, and happier. I couldn't believe that I could find so few people talking about it at that time.

Elevating social health alongside physical and mental health is the way to remedy the three issues I outlined in chapter 1 that have held us back from being as healthy as we can be: most people underestimate the importance of relationships; connection gets lost in the conversation on mental health, when in fact it determines physical health and longevity as well; and we need a positive, asset-focused framework that is inviting, generative, and proactive.

This idea feels so important to me and so urgent for the world that I have dedicated my career to decoding and disseminating it—first with small steps, trying to verify that it truly had merit, then at a jog, writing articles and giving talks, and now, with this book, full-on running.

And I'm no longer alone. In the past few years, Google Search trends for "What is social health" have shot up in the US[1] and worldwide.[2] There are now organizations that herald social health in their mission statements and a growing movement of researchers, nonprofit founders, government leaders, corporate executives, and everyday people around the world championing social health.

This is just the beginning.

After more than ten years of studying, sharing, and shaping these efforts, I feel nothing but optimism for our ability to overcome the challenges that have left so many people feeling disconnected, overly connected, or connected in unfulfilling ways.

I predict that in the next ten to twenty years, building on the momentum and traction thus far, social health will become as pervasive an idea as physical and mental health. In the same way that mental health has risen in prominence, social health will rise. It is the natural next step in our evolution of understanding what it means to be healthy.

This book is meant to spark many more conversations about this topic, not have the final say. I hope people will pick up where I have left off, adding what I've missed, expanding on what I've laid out, and further refining the concept and practice of social health. I hope it grows and spreads its wings from here.

When you close this book and look around you today and each day going forward, I invite you to seize opportunities to enrich your social health, other people's social health, and our collective social health. Those opportunities are everywhere.

Acknowledgments

This journey has given me a long list of thank-you cards to write! Special thanks to the following people in particular:

Esmond, thank you for immediately seeing the potential in my idea and helping me articulate, refine, and bring it to life. Your graciousness and prowess are a joy to work with.

Anna, thank you for believing in me from the start and patiently holding up a lantern to guide me through the fog of writing and editing into the light of publishing my first book.

Thank you to the terrific teams who made the magic happen behind the scenes. I am especially grateful to Erin, Mags, and Vanessa at Aevitas; Chantal, Melinda, Julia, Biz, Aly, Amy, and Judith at HarperOne; Holly, Gabriella, Sarah, John, and Narjas at Little, Brown; and Barbara and Mark at Fortier.

Thank you to everyone I interviewed for generously sharing your expertise and experiences; you inspire me. Thank you to the trusted confidants who provided feedback on earlier drafts and my many wonderful colleagues and collaborators in this work over the years.

Nim, thank you for showing up exactly when I needed you and being my champion, strategist, and, ultimately, friend. Stef, thank you for helping make the beginning of this book ten times better, reassuring me in moments of self-doubt, and being my *anam cara*. Rachel, Katie, and Adam, thank you for your invaluable insights the many times I asked for input. Amy, thank you for your scrupulous eye and thoughtfulness. Eli, thank you for our uplifting conversations.

Mum, thank you for always being there to listen and laugh

together, for your sage writing advice, and for encouraging me to do bold things from a young age. To all my family and friends, thank you for cheering me on and being my cherished sources of social health.

Marcus, thank you for walking down the stairs and into my life. You are my stable foundation, my home, my love. I could not have written this book without your daily support.

Appendix

FURTHER READING

If you enjoyed this book, you may also enjoy my newsletter, where I share new articles, practical tips, events and opportunities, personal reflections, book recommendations, and other resources to help you connect meaningfully. As the idea and practice of social health continuously evolve, this is also where I will highlight new research and emerging trends. You can sign up at www.kasleykillam.com/newsletter.

NOTE

Despite rigorous attention to detail and commitment to accuracy by me and everyone involved with this book, mistakes are possible (if not inevitable!). Please get in touch on my website if you come across any so we can correct them in future editions.

Notes

Introduction: The Future of Health Is Social

1. US Department of Health and Human Services, Office of the US Surgeon General, "Advisory: The Healing Effects of Social Connection," 2023, https://www.hhs.gov/surgeongeneral/priorities/connection/index.html.
2. Daniel A. Cox, "The State of American Friendship: Change, Challenges, and Loss," Survey Center on American Life, June 8, 2021, https://www.americansurveycenter.org/research/the-state-of-american-friendship-change-challenges-and-loss/.
3. US Department of Health and Human Services, Office of the US Surgeon General, "Advisory: The Healing Effects of Social Connection."
4. Aleksandra Sandstrom and Becka A. Alper, "Americans with Higher Education and Income Are More Likely to Be Involved in Community Groups," Pew Research Center, February 22, 2019, https://www.pewresearch.org/short-reads/2019/02/22/americans-with-higher-education-and-income-are-more-likely-to-be-involved-in-community-groups/; Kristen Purcell and Aaron Smith, "The Social Side of the Internet, Section 1: The State of Groups and Voluntary Organizations in America," Pew Research Center, January 18, 2011, https://www.pewresearch.org/internet/2011/01/18/section-1-the-state-of-groups-and-voluntary-organizations-in-america/.
5. Cigna, "Loneliness and the Workplace: 2020 U.S. Report," January 2020, https://www.cigna.com/static/www-cigna-com/docs/about-us/newsroom/studies-and-reports/combatting-loneliness/cigna-2020-loneliness-report.pdf.
6. Gallup Organization, "Gallup Global Emotions 2022," https://img.lalr.co/cms/2022/06/29185719/2022-Gallup-Global-Emotions-Report-2022_compressed.pdf.
7. US Department of Health and Human Services, Office of the US Surgeon General, "Advisory: The Healing Effects of Social Connection."
8. Christina Carrega and Priya Krishnakumar, "Hate Crime Reports in US Surge to the Highest Level in 12 Years, FBI Says," CNN, October 26,

2021, https://www.cnn.com/2021/08/30/us/fbi-report-hate-crimes
-rose-2020/index.html.

9.   Michael Dimock and Richard Wike, "America Is Exceptional in the Nature of Its Political Divide," Pew Research Center, November 13, 2020,
https://www.pewresearch.org/short-reads/2020/11/13/america-is
-exceptional-in-the-nature-of-its-political-divide/.

10. Lee Rainie and Andrew Perrin, "The State of Americans' Trust in Each
Other amid the COVID-19 Pandemic," Pew Research Center, April 6,
2020, https://www.pewresearch.org/short-reads/2020/04/06
/the-state-of-americans-trust-in-each-other-amid-the-covid-19
-pandemic/.

Chapter 1: Redefine What It Means to Be Healthy

1.   Ido Badash et al., "Redefining Health: The Evolution of Health Ideas
from Antiquity to the Era of Value-Based Care," *Cureus* 9, no. 2 (February 9, 2017): e1018, https://doi.org/10.7759/cureus.1018.

2.   K. Michael Cummings and Robert N. Proctor, "The Changing Public
Image of Smoking in the United States: 1964–2014," *Cancer Epidemiology, Biomarkers & Prevention* 23, no. 1 (January 1, 2014): 32–36, https
://doi.org/10.1158/1055-9965.epi-13-0798.

3.   Our World in Data, "Global Child Mortality," 2023, https://ourworld
indata.org/grapher/global-child-mortality-timeseries.

4.   Saloni Dattani et al., "Life Expectancy," Our World in Data, 2013, re-
vised October 2019, https://ourworldindata.org/life-expectancy.

5.   Mandy Erickson, "Alcoholics Anonymous Most Effective Path to
Alcohol Abstinence," Stanford Medicine News Center, March 11, 2020,
https://med.stanford.edu/news/all-news/2020/03/alcoholics
-anonymous-most-effective-path-to-alcohol-abstinence.html.

6.   Lisa F. Berkman and S. Leonard Syme, "Social Networks, Host Resis-
tance, and Mortality: A Nine-Year Follow-up Study of Alameda County
Residents," *American Journal of Epidemiology* 109, no. 2 (February
1979): 186–204, https://doi.org/10.1093/oxfordjournals.aje.a112674.

7.   Jaime Vila, "Social Support and Longevity: Meta-Analysis-Based Evidence and Psychobiological Mechanisms," *Frontiers in Psychology* 12,
art. 717164 (September 13, 2021), https://doi.org/10.3389
/fpsyg.2021.717164.

8.   Fan Wang et al., "A Systematic Review and Meta-Analysis of 90 Cohort
Studies of Social Isolation, Loneliness and Mortality," *Nature Human
Behaviour* 7 (June 2023): 1–13, https://doi.org/10.1038/s41562-023
-01617-6.

9.   Julianne Holt-Lunstad, "The Potential Public Health Relevance of
Social Isolation and Loneliness: Prevalence, Epidemiology, and Risk

Factors," *Public Policy & Aging Report* 27, no. 4 (2017): 127–30, https://doi.org/10.1093/ppar/prx030; Julianne Holt-Lunstad, Theodore F. Robles, and David A. Sbarra, "Advancing Social Connection as a Public Health Priority in the United States," *American Psychologist* 72, no. 6 (2017): 517–30, https://doi.org/10.1037/amp0000103.

10. Jeremy Howick, Paul Kelly, and Mike Kelly, "Establishing a Causal Link Between Social Relationships and Health Using the Bradford Hill Guidelines," *ScienceDirect*, Vol. 8, August 2019, https://www.sciencedirect.com/science/article/pii/S2352827318303501.

11. Sheldon Cohen et al., "Does Hugging Provide Stress-Buffering Social Support? A Study of Susceptibility to Upper Respiratory Infection and Illness," *Psychological Science* 26, no. 2 (2014): 135–47, https://doi.org/10.1177/0956797614559284.

12. Sheldon Cohen et al., "Social Ties and Susceptibility to the Common Cold," *Journal of the American Medical Association* 277, no. 24 (1997): 1940, https://doi.org/10.1001/jama.1997.03540480040036.

13. Nicole K. Valtorta et al., "Loneliness and Social Isolation as Risk Factors for Coronary Heart Disease and Stroke: Systematic Review and Meta-Analysis of Longitudinal Observational Studies," *Heart* 102, no. 13 (2016): 1009–16, https://doi.org/10.1136/heartjnl-2015-308790.

14. My Health My Community, "Social Connection and Health," March 2018, https://myhealthmycommunity.org/wp-content/uploads/2019/05/MHMC_SocialConnections_web.pdf.

15. Robert Waldinger, "What Makes a Good Life? Lessons from the Longest Study on Happiness," TEDxBeaconStreet video, 12:38, November 2015, https://www.ted.com/talks/robert_waldinger_what_makes_a_good_life_lessons_from_the_longest_study_on_happiness.

16. Joni L. Strom and Leonard E. Egede, "The Impact of Social Support on Outcomes in Adult Patients with Type 2 Diabetes: A Systematic Review," *Current Diabetes Reports* 12, no. 6 (2012): 769–81, https://doi.org/10.1007/s11892-012-0317-0.

17. Henk A. van Dam et al., "Social Support in Diabetes: A Systematic Review of Controlled Intervention Studies," *Patient Education and Counseling* 59, no. 1 (October 2005): 1–12, https://doi.org/10.1016/j.pec.2004.11.001.

18. Bina Nausheen et al., "Social Support and Cancer Progression: A Systematic Review," *Journal of Psychosomatic Research* 67, no. 5 (November 2009): 403–15, https://doi.org/10.1016/j.jpsychores.2008.12.012.

19. Bert N. Uchino et al., "Social Support, Social Integration, and Inflammatory Cytokines: A Meta-Analysis," *Health Psychology* 37, no. 5 (2018): 462–71, https://doi.org/10.1037/hea0000594.

20. Erica A. Hornstein, Michael S. Fanselow, and Naomi I. Eisenberger, "A Safe Haven: Investigating Social-Support Figures as Prepared Safety

Stimuli," *Psychological Science* 27, no. 8 (2016): 1051–60, https://doi .org/10.1177/0956797616646580.

21.   Livia Tomova et al., "Acute Social Isolation Evokes Midbrain Craving Responses Similar to Hunger," *Nature Neuroscience* 23, no. 12 (2020): 1597–1605, https://doi.org/10.1038/s41593-020-00742-z.

22.   Naomi I. Eisenberger, "The Pain of Social Disconnection: Examining the Shared Neural Underpinnings of Physical and Social Pain," *Nature Reviews Neuroscience* 13, no. 6 (2012): 421–34, https://doi.org/10.1038 /nrn3231.

23.   M. Robin DiMatteo, "Social Support and Patient Adherence to Medical Treatment: A Meta-Analysis," *Health Psychology* 23, no. 2 (2004): 207–18, https://doi.org/10.1037/0278-6133.23.2.207.

24.   Tamsyn Hawken, Julie Turner-Cobb, and Julie Barnett, "Coping and Adjustment in Caregivers: A Systematic Review," *Health Psychology Open* 5, no. 2 (2018), https://doi.org/10.1177/2055102918810659.

25.   Andrew Stickley and Ai Koyanagi, "Loneliness, Common Mental Disorders and Suicidal Behavior: Findings from a General Population Survey," *Journal of Affective Disorders* 197 (June 2016): 81–87, https:// doi.org/10.1016/j.jad.2016.02.054.

26.   Ziggi Ivan Santini et al., "The Association Between Social Relation- ships and Depression: A Systematic Review," *Journal of Affective Disor- ders* 175 (2015): 53–65, https://doi.org/10.1016/j.jad.2014.12.049.

27.   John T. Cacioppo, Louise C. Hawkley, and Ronald A. Thisted, "Per- ceived Social Isolation Makes Me Sad: 5-Year Cross-Lagged Analyses of Loneliness and Depressive Symptomatology in the Chicago Health, Aging, and Social Relations Study," *Psychology and Aging* 25, no. 2 (2010): 453–63, https://doi.org/10.1037/a0017216.

28.   Tarja Heponiemi et al., "The Longitudinal Effects of Social Support and Hostility on Depressive Tendencies," *Social Science & Medicine* 63, no. 5 (September 2006): 1374–82, https://doi.org/10.1016 /j.socscimed.2006.03.036.

29.   Alexander K. Saeri et al., "Social Connectedness Improves Public Mental Health: Investigating Bidirectional Relationships in the New Zealand Attitudes and Values Survey," *Australian & New Zealand Journal of Psychiatry* 52, no. 4 (2017): 365–74, https://doi.org/10.1177 /0004867417723990.

30.   Jisca S. Kuiper et al., "Social Relationships and Risk of Dementia: A Systematic Review and Meta-Analysis of Longitudinal Cohort Stud- ies," *Ageing Research Reviews* 22 (July 2015): 39–57, https://doi.org /10.1016/j.arr.2015.04.006.

31.   Carlo Lazzari and Marco Rabottini, "COVID-19, Loneliness, Social Isolation and Risk of Dementia in Older People: A Systematic Review and Meta-Analysis of the Relevant Literature," *International Journal of*

Psychiatry in Clinical Practice 26, no. 2 (2021): 1–12, https://doi.org /10.1080/13651501.2021.1959616.

32. Karynna Okabe-Miyamoto and Sonja Lyubomirsky, "Social Connection and Well-Being During COVID-19," chap. 6 in *World Happiness Report 2021*, edited by John F. Helliwell et al. (New York: Sustainable Development Solutions Network, 2021), https://worldhappiness .report/ed/2021/social-connection-and-well-being-during-covid-19/.

33. Shimon Saphire-Bernstein and Shelley E. Taylor, "Close Relationships and Happiness," in *Oxford Handbook of Happiness*, edited by Ilona Boniwell, Susan A. David, and Amanda Conley Ayers, 821–33 (Oxford: Oxford Univ. Press, 2013), https://doi.org/10.1093/oxfordhb /9780199557257.013.0060.

34. S. Alexander Haslam et al., "Social Cure, What Social Cure? The Propensity to Underestimate the Importance of Social Factors for Health," *Social Science & Medicine* 198 (February 2018): 14–21, https:// doi.org/10.1016/j.socscimed.2017.12.020.

35. Andy Proctor, "The Best Thing to Improve Your Health in 2023," *Psychology Today* (blog post), February 28, 2023, https://www.psychology today.com/us/blog/more-happy-life/202302/the-best-thing-to -improve-your-health-in-2023.

36. Bianca DiJulio, "Loneliness and Social Isolation in the United States, the United Kingdom, and Japan: An International Survey," KFF, August 30, 2018, https://www.kff.org/mental-health/report/loneliness -and-social-isolation-in-the-united-states-the-united-kingdom-and -japan-an-international-survey.

37. Lydia Saad, "COVID-19 Still Widely Named as Biggest U.S. Health Problem," Gallup, November 30, 2021, https://news.gallup.com /poll/357707/covid-widely-named-biggest-health-problem.aspx.

38. Richard Weissbourd et al., "Loneliness in America: How the Pandemic Has Deepened an Epidemic of Loneliness and What We Can Do About It," Making Caring Common Project, Harvard Graduate School of Education, February 2021, https://mcc.gse.harvard.edu/reports /loneliness-in-america.

39. Lynda Flowers et al., "Medicare Spends More on Socially Isolated Older Adults," AARP Public Policy Institute, November 2017, https:// www.aarp.org/content/dam/aarp/ppi/2017/10/medicare-spends -more-on-socially-isolated-older-adults.pdf; Cigna, "Loneliness and Its Impact on the American Workplace," March 2020, https://www .cigna.com/static/www-cigna-com/docs/about-us/newsroom/studies -and-reports/combatting-loneliness/loneliness-and-its-impact-on -the-american-workplace.pdf.

40. Peter Gibbon, "Martin Seligman and the Rise of Positive Psychology,"

Humanities 41, no. 3 (Summer 2020), https://www.neh.gov/article
/martin-seligman-and-rise-positive-psychology.

Chapter 2: Demystify Your Relationships

1. Peter Kitchen, Allison Williams, and James Chowhan, "Sense of Community Belonging and Health in Canada: A Regional Analysis," *Social Indicators Research* 107, no. 1 (2012): 103–26, https://doi.org/10.1007/s11205-011-9830-9.
2. Sachiko Inoue et al., "Social Cohesion and Mortality: A Survival Analysis of Older Adults in Japan," *American Journal of Public Health* 103, no. 12 (2013): e60–66, https://doi.org/10.2105/ajph.2013.301311.
3. Tegan Cruwys et al., "Social Group Memberships Protect Against Future Depression, Alleviate Depression Symptoms and Prevent Depression Relapse," *Social Science & Medicine* 98 (December 2013): 179–86, https://doi.org/10.1016/j.socscimed.2013.09.013.
4. Rosemary Blieszner and Karen A. Roberto, "Friendship Across the Life Span: Reciprocity in Individual and Relationship Development," in *Growing Together: Personal Relationships Across the Life Span*, edited by Frieder R. Lang and Karen L. Fingerman, 159–82 (Cambridge, UK: Cambridge Univ. Press, 2004).
5. Harvard University, Center on the Developing Child, "Resilience," n.d., accessed March 2023, https://developingchild.harvard.edu/science/key-concepts/resilience/.
6. Wändi Bruine de Bruin, Andrew M. Parker, and JoNell Strough, "Age Differences in Reported Social Networks and Well-Being," *Psychology and Aging* 35, no. 2 (2020): 159–68, https://doi.org/10.1037/pag0000415.
7. Kiffer G. Card et al., "Evidence Brief: How Many Friends Do You Need?," Canadian Alliance for Social Connection and Health, 2022, https://static1.squarespace.com/static/60283c2e174c122f8ebe0f39/t/645a88655583045704102e40/1683654757592/CSCG_Evidence+Brief_Number+of+Friends.pdf.
8. Cheryl L. Carmichael, Harry T. Reis, and Paul R. Duberstein, "In Your 20s It's Quantity, in Your 30s It's Quality: The Prognostic Value of Social Activity Across 30 Years of Adulthood," *Psychology and Aging* 30, no. 1 (2015): 95–105, https://doi.org/10.1037/pag0000014.

Chapter 3: Reveal Your Social Health Style

1. American Cancer Society, "Survival Rates for Pancreatic Cancer," March 2, 2023, https://www.cancer.org/cancer/types/pancreatic-cancer/detection-diagnosis-staging/survival-rates.html.
2. Jessie Sun, Kelci Harris, and Simine Vazire, "Is Well-Being Associated

with the Quantity and Quality of Social Interactions?," *Journal of Personality and Social Psychology* 119, no. 6 (2020): 1478–96, https://doi.org/10.1037/pspp0000272.

3. Kiffer G. Card and Pete Bombaci, "Social Connection in Canada: Preliminary Results from the 2021 Canadian Social Connection Survey," GenWell Project, 2021, https://genwellproject.org/wp-content/uploads/2021/07/Social-Connection-in-Canada_Release-1.pdf.

4. Kiffer G. Card et al., "Evidence Brief: How Much Social Time Do We Need?," Canadian Alliance for Social Connection and Health, 2022, https://static1.squarespace.com/static/60283c2e174c122f8ebe0f39/t/64886fce584f4410556959e2/1686663119192/CSCG_Evidence+Brief_Social+Time.pdf.

5. Canadian Alliance for Social Connection and Health, "Social Connection Guidelines," n.d., accessed March 2023, https://casch.org/guidelines.

6. Joyce J. Slater and Adriana N. Mudryj, "Are We Really 'Eating Well with Canada's Food Guide'?," *BMC Public Health* 18, no. 1 (2018), https://doi.org/10.1186/s12889-018-5540-4.

7. Hanne K. Collins et al., "Relational Diversity in Social Portfolios Predicts Well-Being," *Proceedings of the National Academy of Sciences* 119, no. 43 (October 17, 2022), https://www.hbs.edu/faculty/Pages/item.aspx?num=62955.

8. Eran Shor, David J. Roelfs, and Tamar Yogev, "The Strength of Family Ties: A Meta-Analysis and Meta-Regression of Self-Reported Social Support and Mortality," *Social Networks* 35, no. 4 (October 2013): 626–38, https://doi.org/10.1016/j.socnet.2013.08.004.

9. William J. Chopik, "Associations Among Relational Values, Support, Health, and Well-Being Across the Adult Lifespan," *Personal Relationships* 24, no. 2 (2017): 408–22, https://doi.org/10.1111/pere.12187.

10. R. Weiss, "The Provisions of Social Relationships," in *Doing Unto Others*, edited by Z. Rubin, 17–26 (Englewood Cliffs, NJ: Prentice Hall, 1974).

11. Esther Perel, "The Secret to Desire in a Long-Term Relationship," TEDSalon NY video, 18:54, February 2013, https://www.ted.com/talks/esther_perel_the_secret_to_desire_in_a_long_term_relationship.

12. Robert G. Wood, Brian Goesling, and Sarah Avellar, "The Effects of Marriage on Health: A Synthesis of Recent Research Evidence," US Department of Health and Human Services, June 19, 2007, https://www.healthymarriageinfo.org/wp-content/uploads/1164.pdf.

13. Lamberto Manzoli et al., "Marital Status and Mortality in the Elderly: A Systematic Review and Meta-Analysis," *Social Science & Medicine* 64, no. 1 (2007): 77–94, https://doi.org/10.1016/j.socscimed.2006.08.031.

14. Deborah Carr et al., "Happy Marriage, Happy Life? Marital Quality

and Subjective Well-Being in Later Life," *Journal of Marriage and Family* 76, no. 5 (October 2014): 930–48, https://doi.org/10.1111/jomf.12133.

15. Toshihide Iwase et al., "Do Bonding and Bridging Social Capital Have Differential Effects on Self-Rated Health? A Community Based Study in Japan," *Journal of Epidemiology and Community Health* 66, no. 6 (2012): 557–62, https://doi.org/10.1136/jech.2010.115592.

16. Kristin Neff, "Self-Compassion," Self-Compassion, n.d., accessed March 2023, https://self-compassion.org/.

17. Christopher M. Masi et al., "A Meta-Analysis of Interventions to Reduce Loneliness," *Personality and Social Psychology Review* 15, no. 3 (2011): 219–66, https://doi.org/10.1177/1088868310377394.

18. Kasley Killam, "Bridging the Intergenerational Divide," *Medium* (blog), December 30, 2018, https://medium.com/world-economic-forum-global-shapers-san-francisco/bridging-the-intergenerational-divide-5ee500025774.

19. Elizabeth Brondolo et al., "Racism and Social Capital: The Implications for Social and Physical Well-Being," *Journal of Social Issues* 68, no. 2 (2012): 358–84, https://doi.org/10.1111/j.1540-4560.2012.01752.x.

20. Elizabeth A. Pascoe and Laura Smart Richman, "Perceived Discrimination and Health: A Meta-Analytic Review," *Psychological Bulletin* 135, no. 4 (2009): 531–54, https://doi.org/10.1037/a0016059.

21. Lydia Saad, "COVID-19 Still Widely Named as Biggest U.S. Health Problem," Gallup, November 30, 2021, https://news.gallup.com/poll/357707/covid-widely-named-biggest-health-problem.aspx.

22. Lydia Saad, "People of Color Help Boost Nation's Bleak Race Ratings," Gallup, February 9, 2022, https://news.gallup.com/poll/389540/people-color-help-boost-nations-bleak-race-ratings.aspx.

23. Julianne Holt-Lunstad and Bert N. Uchino, "Social Ambivalence and Disease (SAD): A Theoretical Model Aimed at Understanding the Health Implications of Ambivalent Relationships," *Perspectives on Psychological Science* 14, no. 6 (2019): 941–66, https://doi.org/10.1177/1745691619861392.

24. Nielsen, "The Nielsen Total Audience Report: August 2020," August 2020, https://www.nielsen.com/insights/2020/the-nielsen-total-audience-report-august-2020/.

25. Brooke Auxier and Monica Anderson, "Social Media Use in 2021," Pew Research Center, April 7, 2021, https://www.pewresearch.org/internet/2021/04/07/social-media-use-in-2021/.

26. Katherine Schaeffer, "Most U.S. Teens Who Use Cellphones Do It to Pass Time, Connect with Others, Learn New Things," Pew Research Center, August 23, 2019, https://www.pewresearch.org/short-reads/2019/08/23/most-u-s-teens-who-use-cellphones-do-it-to-pass-time-connect-with-others-learn-new-things/.

27. Monica Anderson and Jingjing Jiang, "Teens' Social Media Habits and Experiences," Pew Research Center, November 28, 2018, https://www .pewresearch.org/internet/2018/11/28/teens-social-media-habits -and-experiences/.

28. Melissa G. Hunt et al., "No More FOMO: Limiting Social Media Decreases Loneliness and Depression," *Journal of Social and Clinical Psychology* 37, no. 10 (2018): 751–68, https://doi.org/10.1521 /jscp.2018.37.10.751.

29. Emily B. O'Day and Richard G. Heimberg, "Social Media Use, Social Anxiety, and Loneliness: A Systematic Review," *Computers in Human Behavior Reports* 3 (January–July 2021): 100070, https://doi.org /10.1016/j.chbr.2021.100070.

30. Roger O'Sullivan et al., "Impact of the COVID-19 Pandemic on Loneliness and Social Isolation: A Multi-Country Study," *International Journal of Environmental Research and Public Health* 18, no. 19 (2021): 9982, https://doi.org/10.3390/ijerph18199982.

31. AARP Foundation and United Health Foundation, "The Pandemic Effect: A Social Isolation Report," Connect2Affect.org, October 6, 2020, https://connect2affect.org/wp-content/uploads/2020/10/The -Pandemic-Effect-A-Social-Isolation-Report-AARP-Foundation.pdf.

32. Richard Weissbourd et al., "Loneliness in America: How the Pandemic Has Deepened an Epidemic of Loneliness and What We Can Do About It," Making Caring Common Project, Harvard Graduate School of Education, February 2021, https://mcc.gse.harvard.edu/reports /loneliness-in-america.

33. Gabriele Prati and Anthony D. Mancini, "The Psychological Impact of COVID-19 Pandemic Lockdowns: A Review and Meta-Analysis of Longitudinal Studies and Natural Experiments," *Psychological Medicine* 51, no. 2 (2021): 201–11, https://doi.org/10.1017/s0033291721000015.

34. Mareike Ernst et al., "Loneliness Before and During the COVID-19 Pandemic: A Systematic Review with Meta-Analysis," *American Psychologist* 77, no. 5 (2022): 660–77, https://doi.org/10.1037 /amp0001005.

35. Martina Luchetti et al., "The Trajectory of Loneliness in Response to COVID-19," *American Psychologist* 75, no. 7 (2020): 897–908, https:// doi.org/10.1037/amp0000690.

36. American Lung Association, "Overall Tobacco Trends," n.d., accessed March 2023, https://www.lung.org/research/trends-in-lung-disease /tobacco-trends-brief/overall-tobacco-trends.

37. Kamal Fatehi, Jennifer L. Priestley, and Gita Taasoobshirazi, "The Expanded View of Individualism and Collectivism: One, Two, or Four Dimensions?," *International Journal of Cross Cultural Management* 20, no. 1 (2020): 7–24, https://doi.org/10.1177/1470595820913077.

38. Manuela Barreto et al., "Loneliness Around the World: Age, Gender, and Cultural Differences in Loneliness," *Personality and Individual Differences* 169 (2021): 110066, https://doi.org/10.1016/j.paid.2020.110066.

39. Mie Kito, Masaki Yuki, and Robert Thomson, "Relational Mobility and Close Relationships: A Socioecological Approach to Explain Cross-Cultural Differences," *Personal Relationships* 24, no. 1 (March 2017): 114–30, https://doi.org/10.1111/pere.12174.

40. Johannes Beller and Adina Wagner, "Loneliness and Health: The Moderating Effect of Cross-Cultural Individualism/Collectivism," *Journal of Aging and Health* 32, no. 10 (2020): 1516–27, https://doi.org/10.1177/0898264320943336.

41. Esteban Ortiz-Ospina, "The Rise of Living Alone: How One-Person Households Are Becoming Increasingly Common Around the World," Our World in Data, December 10, 2019, https://ourworldindata.org/living-alone.

Chapter 4: Make Social Health a Priority

1. John M. Darley and C. Daniel Batson, "'From Jerusalem to Jericho': A Study of Situational and Dispositional Variables in Helping Behavior," *Journal of Personality and Social Psychology* 27, no. 1 (1973): 100–108, https://doi.org/10.1037/h0034449.

2. Patrick van Kessel, "How Americans Feel About the Satisfactions and Stresses of Modern Life," Pew Research Center, February 5, 2020, https://www.pewresearch.org/short-reads/2020/02/05/how-americans-feel-about-the-satisfactions-and-stresses-of-modern-life/.

3. Gilliam M. Sandstrom and Elizabeth W. Dunn, "Is Efficiency Overrated? Minimal Social Interactions Lead to Belonging and Positive Affect," *Social Psychological and Personality Science* 5, no. 4 (2014): 437–42, https://doi.org/10.1177/1948550613502990.

Chapter 5: Strengthen Your Social Muscles

1. Jeffrey A. Hall, "How Many Hours Does It Take to Make a Friend?," *Journal of Social and Personal Relationships* 36, no. 4 (2019): 1278–96, https://doi.org/10.1177/0265407518761225.

2. Dawn C. Carr et al., "Does Becoming a Volunteer Attenuate Loneliness Among Recently Widowed Older Adults?," *Journals of Gerontology: Series B* 73, no. 3 (March 2018): 501–10, https://doi.org/10.1093/geronb/gbx092.

3. Nancy Morrow-Howell et al., "Effects of Volunteering on the Well-Being of Older Adults," *Journals of Gerontology: Series B* 58, no. 3 (May 2003): S137–45, https://doi.org/10.1093/geronb/58.3.s137.

4.   David A. Preece et al., "Loneliness and Emotion Regulation," *Personality and Individual Differences* 180 (October 2021): 110974, https://doi .org/10.1016/j.paid.2021.110974.

5.   Eden Litt et al., "What Are Meaningful Social Interactions in Today's Media Landscape? A Cross-Cultural Survey," *Social Media + Society* 6, no. 3 (2020): 205630512094288, https://doi.org/10.1177 /2056305120942888.

6.   Nancy L. Collins and Lynn Carol Miller, "Self-Disclosure and Liking: A Meta-Analytic Review," *Psychological Bulletin* 116, no. 3 (1994): 457–75, https://doi.org/10.1037/0033-2909.116.3.457.

7.   Emily Towner et al., "Revealing the Self in a Digital World: A Systematic Review of Adolescent Online and Offline Self-Disclosure," *Current Opinion in Psychology* 45 (June 2022): 101309, https://doi.org/10.1016 /j.copsyc.2022.101309.

8.   Sara B. Algoe, Jonathan Haidt, and Shelly L. Gable, "Beyond Reciprocity: Gratitude and Relationships in Everyday Life," *Emotion* 8, no. 3 (2008): 425–29, https://doi.org/10.1037/1528-3542.8.3.425.

9.   Amie M. Gordon, "Gratitude Is for Lovers," *Greater Good Magazine*, February 5, 2013, https://greatergood.berkeley.edu/article/item /gratitude_is_for_lovers.

10.   Sara B. Algoe, "Find, Remind, and Bind: The Functions of Gratitude in Everyday Relationships," *Social and Personality Psychology Compass* 6, no. 6 (June 2012): 455–69, https://doi.org/10.1111/j.1751-9004.2012 .00439.x.

11.   Summer Allen, "The Science of Gratitude," Greater Good Science Center, University of California, Berkeley, May 2018, https://ggsc .berkeley.edu/images/uploads/GGSC-JTF_White_Paper-Gratitude -FINAL.pdf.

12.   Robert Emmons, "Why Gratitude Is Good," *Greater Good Magazine*, November 16, 2010, https://greatergood.berkeley.edu/article/item /why_gratitude_is_good.

13.   Lisa C. Walsh et al., "What Is the Optimal Way to Give Thanks? Comparing the Effects of Gratitude Expressed Privately, One-to-One via Text, or Publicly on Social Media," *Affective Science* 4 (March 2023): 82–91, https://doi.org/10.1007/s42761-022-00150-5.

14.   Nextdoor, "About Nextdoor," n.d., accessed March 2023, https://about .nextdoor.com/.

15.   Nextdoor, "Global Study Finds Knowing as Few as 6 Neighbors Reduces the Likelihood of Loneliness," December 2, 2020, https://about .nextdoor.com/global-study-finds-knowing-as-few-as-6-neighbors -reduces-the-likelihood-of-loneliness/.

16.   Oliver Scott Curry et al., "Happy to Help? A Systematic Review and Meta-Analysis of the Effects of Performing Acts of Kindness on the

Well-Being of the Actor," *Journal of Experimental Social Psychology* 76 (May 2018): 320–29, https://doi.org/10.1016/j.jesp.2018.02.014.

17. Lee Rowland and Oliver Scott Curry, "A Range of Kindness Activities Boost Happiness," *Journal of Social Psychology* 159, no. 3 (2018): 340–43, https://doi.org/10.1080/00224545.2018.1469461.

18. Elizabeth W. Dunn, Lara B. Aknin, and Michael I. Norton, "Spending Money on Others Promotes Happiness," *Science* 319, no. 5870 (March 21, 2008): 1687–88, https://doi.org/10.1126/science.1150952.

19. Priya Parker, "The Art of Guesting During Festive Season," *Priya Parker* (blog), November 30, 2022, https://www.priyaparker.com/art-of-gathering-newsletter/the-art-of-guesting-during-festive-season.

20. Allied Market Research, "Global Mental Health Market: Opportunities and Forecast, 2021–2030," July 2021, https://www.alliedmarket research.com/mental-health-market-A11770.

21. Kate Jopling, "Promising Approaches to Reducing Loneliness and Isolation in Later Life," Age UK and Campaign to End Loneliness, January 2015, https://www.campaigntoendloneliness.org/wp-content/uploads/Promising-approaches-to-reducing-loneliness-and-isolation-in-later-life.pdf.

22. NHS England, "Social Prescribing," n.d., accessed March 2023, https://www.england.nhs.uk/personalisedcare/social-prescribing/.

23. Hamaad Khan et al., "Social Prescribing Around the World," National Academy for Social Prescribing, 2023, https://socialprescribingacademy.org.uk/media/4lbdy5ip/social-prescribing-around-the-world.pdf.

24. G. Y. Reinhardt, D. Vidovic, and C. Hammerton, "Understanding Loneliness: A Systematic Review of the Impact of Social Prescribing Initiatives on Loneliness," *Perspectives in Public Health* 141, no. 4 (2021): 204–13, https://doi.org/10.1177/1757913920967040.

25. Blerina Kellezi et al., "The Social Cure of Social Prescribing: A Mixed-Methods Study on the Benefits of Social Connectedness on Quality and Effectiveness of Care Provision," *BMJ Open* 9, no. 11 (2019): e033137, https://doi.org/10.1136/bmjopen-2019-033137.

Chapter 6: Take One Small Step for You, One Giant Leap for Social Health

1. Maciej Banach et al., "The Association Between Daily Step Count and All-Cause and Cardiovascular Mortality: A Meta-Analysis," *European Journal of Preventive Cardiology* (August 2023), https://doi.org/10.1093/eurjpc/zwad229.

2. Gretchen Reynolds, "Exercise for 3 Minutes, Every Half-Hour, to Counter the Ill Effects of Sitting," *New York Times*, September 8, 2021, https://www.nytimes.com/2021/09/08/well/move/work-breaks-sitting-metabolic-health.html.

3.   Marla Reicks et al., "Frequency of Eating Alone Is Associated with Adolescent Dietary Intake, Perceived Food-Related Parenting Practices and Weight Status: Cross-Sectional Family Life, Activity, Sun, Health, and Eating (FLASHE) Study Results," *Public Health Nutrition* 22, no. 9 (2019): 1555–66, https://doi.org/10.1017/s1368980019000107.

4.   Jean M. Twenge et al., "Worldwide Increases in Adolescent Loneliness," *Journal of Adolescence* 93, no. 1 (December 2021), https://doi.org/10.1016/j.adolescence.2021.06.006.

5.   Daniel A. Cox, "The Childhood Loneliness of Generation Z," Survey Center on American Life, April 4, 2022, https://www.americansurveycenter.org/the-lonely-childhood-of-generation-z/.

6.   Ryu Takizawa, Barbara Maughan, and Louise Arseneault, "Adult Health Outcomes of Childhood Bullying Victimization: Evidence from a Five-Decade Longitudinal British Birth Cohort," *American Journal of Psychiatry* 171, no. 7 (2014): 777–84, https://doi.org/10.1176/appi.ajp.2014.13101401.

7.   World Health Organization, "Coming of Age: Adolescent Health," n.d., accessed March 2023, https://www.who.int/news-room/spotlight/coming-of-age-adolescent-health.

8.   Carrie L. Masten et al., "Neural Correlates of Social Exclusion During Adolescence: Understanding the Distress of Peer Rejection," *Social Cognitive and Affective Neuroscience* 4, no. 2 (June 2009): 143–57, https://doi.org/10.1093/scan/nsp007.

9.   Peggy J. Liu et al., "The Surprise of Reaching Out: Appreciated More than We Think," *Journal of Personality and Social Psychology* 124, no. 4 (2023): 754–71, https://doi.org/10.1037/pspi0000402.

10.   James A. Dungan, David M. Munguia Gomez, and Nicholas Epley, "Too Reluctant to Reach Out: Receiving Social Support Is More Positive than Expressers Expect," *Psychological Science* 33, no. 8 (2022): 1300–1312, https://doi.org/10.1177/09567976221082942.

11.   Amit Kumar and Nicholas Epley, "A Little Good Goes an Unexpectedly Long Way: Underestimating the Positive Impact of Kindness on Recipients," *Journal of Experimental Psychology: General* 152, no. 1 (2023): 236–52, https://doi.org/10.1037/xge0001271.

12.   Amit Kumar and Nicholas Epley, "Undervaluing Gratitude: Expressers Misunderstand the Consequences of Showing Appreciation," *Psychological Science* 29, no. 9 (2018): 1423–35, https://doi.org/10.1177/0956797618772506.

13.   Maninder K. Kahlon et al., "Effect of Layperson-Delivered, Empathy-Focused Program of Telephone Calls on Loneliness, Depression, and Anxiety Among Adults During the COVID-19 Pandemic: A Randomized Clinical Trial," *JAMA Psychiatry* 78, no. 6 (2021): 616–22, https://doi.org/10.1001/jamapsychiatry.2021.0113.

14. Survey Center on American Life, "Few Gen Zers Grew Up Having Family Dinners," February 9, 2022, https://www.americansurveycenter .org/featured_data/few-gen-zers-grew-up-having-family-dinners.

15. Anne Fishel, "Science Says: Eat with Your Kids," The Conversation, January 9, 2015, https://theconversation.com/science-says-eat-with -your-kids-34573.

Chapter 7: Think Like a Scientist, Even If You're Not One

1. Daniel A. Cox, "Men's Social Circles Are Shrinking," Survey Center on American Life, June 29, 2021, https://www.americansurveycenter .org/why-mens-social-circles-are-shrinking/.

2. Sarah Young, "Millions of British Men Suffering from 'Silent Epidemic' of Loneliness, Says Jo Cox Commission." *Independent,* May 4, 2017, https://www.independent.co.uk/life-style/british-men-peak -loneliness-millions-35-year-old-males-silent-epidemic-jo-cox -commission-spotlight-a7717061.html.

3. Linda Foettinger et al., "The Role of Community-Based Men's Sheds in Health Promotion for Older Men: A Mixed-Methods Systematic Review," *American Journal of Men's Health* 16, no. 2 (March–April 2022), https://doi.org/10.1177/15579883221084490.

4. Erica J. Boothby et al., "The Liking Gap in Conversations: Do People Like Us More than We Think?," *Psychological Science* 29, no. 11 (2018): 1742–56, https://doi.org/10.1177/0956797618783714.

5. Marisa G. Franco (@drmarisagfranco), "1 Tip for Making Friends as an Adult," Instagram video, April 20, 2022, https://www.instagram .com/p/CckbKv1AbR5/.

6. Nikki Forrester, "Fed Up and Burnt Out: 'Quiet Quitting' Hits Academia," *Nature* 615 (March 2023): 751–53, https://doi.org/10.1038 /d41586-023-00633-w.

Chapter 8: Build Community Where You Live

1. Camille Arnodin, "Résilience, convivialité et solidarités de proximité," La 27e Région, 2022, https://www.la27eregion.fr/wp-content /uploads/sites/2/2022/04/Resultats-enquete-Resilience-convivialite -et-solidarites-de-proximite-Synthese-Ville-de-Paris-Mars-2022.pdf.

2. Soumya Mazumdar et al., "The Built Environment and Social Capital: A Systematic Review," *Environment and Behavior* 50, no. 2 (2017): 119–58, https://doi.org/10.1177/0013916516687343.

3. Kasley Killam and Ichiro Kawachi, "Social Capital and Community Design," in *Making Healthy Places: Designing and Building for Well-Being, Equity, and Sustainability,* 2nd ed., edited by Nisha Botchwey, Andrew L. Dannenberg, and Howard Frumkin, 139 (Washington, DC: Island Press, 2022).

4. Lydia Anderson et al., "Share of One-Person Households More than Tripled from 1940 to 2020," US Census Bureau, June 8, 2023, https://www.census.gov/library/stories/2023/06/more-than-a-quarter-all-households-have-one-person.html.

5. Daolin Wu, Fuwei Liu, and Shan Huang, "Assessment of the Relationship Between Living Alone and the Risk of Depression Based on Longitudinal Studies: A Systematic Review and Meta-Analysis," *Frontiers in Psychiatry* 13 (August 30, 2022), https://doi.org/10.3389/fpsyt.2022.954857; Roopal Desai et al., "Living Alone and Risk of Dementia: A Systematic Review and Meta-Analysis," *Ageing Research Reviews* 62 (September 2020): 101122, https://doi.org/10.1016/j.arr.2020.101122.

6. Christos A. Makridis and Cary Wu, "How Social Capital Helps Communities Weather the COVID-19 Pandemic," *PLoS ONE* 16, no. 1 (2021): e0245135, https://doi.org/10.1371/journal.pone.0245135.

7. Alina Kristin Bartscher et al., "Social Capital and the Spread of COVID-19: Insights from European Countries," *Journal of Health Economics* 80 (December 2021): 102531, https://doi.org/10.1016/j.jhealeco.2021.102531.

8. Rebecca Adler-Nissen, Sune Lehmann, and Andreas Roepstorff, "Denmark's Hard Lessons About Trust and the Pandemic," *New York Times*, November 14, 2021, https://www.nytimes.com/2021/11/14/opinion/denmark-trust-covid-vaccine.html.

9. Madeline Drexler, "The Unlikeliest Pandemic Success Story," *Atlantic*, February 10, 2021, https://www.theatlantic.com/international/archive/2021/02/coronavirus-pandemic-bhutan/617976/.

10. Kenneth Pletcher and John P. Rafferty, "Japan Earthquake and Tsunami of 2011," *Encyclopedia Britannica*, November 2, 2023, https://www.britannica.com/event/Japan-earthquake-and-tsunami-of-2011.

11. Hiroyuki Hikichi et al., "Community-Level Social Capital and Cognitive Decline After a Natural Disaster: A Natural Experiment from the 2011 Great East Japan Earthquake and Tsunami," *Social Science & Medicine* 257 (July 2020): 111981, https://doi.org/10.1016/j.socscimed.2018.09.057.

12. Karen Feldscher, "Social Connections Boost Resilience Among Elderly After Disaster," Harvard T.H. Chan School of Public Health, October 8, 2019, https://www.hsph.harvard.edu/news/features/social-connections-boost-resilience-among-elderly-after-disaster/.

Chapter 9: Nurture Connections at Work and Online

1. Cigna, "Loneliness and Its Impact on the American Workplace," March 2020, https://www.cigna.com/static/www-cigna-com/docs/about-us

/newsroom/studies-and-reports/combatting-loneliness/loneliness
-and-its-impact-on-the-american-workplace.pdf.

2. Statista, "Average Daily Time Spent Using the Internet by Online Users
    Worldwide from 3rd Quarter 2015 to 2nd Quarter 2023," 2023, https://
    www.statista.com/statistics/1380282/daily-time-spent-online
    -global/.

3. Statista, "Daily Time Spent on Social Networking by Internet Users
    Worldwide from 2012 to 2023," 2022, https://www.statista.com
    /statistics/433871/daily-social-media-usage-worldwide/.

4. Tom Rath and Jim Harter, "Your Friends and Your Social Well-Being,"
    Gallup Business Journal, August 19, 2010, https://news.gallup.com
    /businessjournal/127043/friends-social-wellbeing.aspx.

5. Cigna, "Loneliness and Its Impact on the American Workplace," March
    2020, https://www.cigna.com/static/www-cigna-com/docs/about-us
    /newsroom/studies-and-reports/combatting-loneliness/loneliness
    -and-its-impact-on-the-american-workplace.pdf.

6. Ernst & Young, "New EY Consulting Survey Confirms 90% of US
    Workers Believe Empathetic Leadership Leads to Higher Job Satisfac-
    tion and 79% Agree It Decreases Employee Turnover," PR Newswire,
    October 14, 2021, https://www.prnewswire.com/news-releases
    /new-ey-consulting-survey-confirms-90-of-us-workers-believe
    -empathetic-leadership-leads-to-higher-job-satisfaction-and-79
    -agree-it-decreases-employee-turnover-301397246.html.

7. Catherine Fisher, "LinkedIn Study Reveals Work BFFs Make Us Hap-
    pier at the Office," *LinkedIn Official Blog*, July 8, 2014, https://blog
    .linkedin.com/2014/07/08/work-bffs.

8. Julia Rozovsky, "The Five Keys to a Successful Google Team," *Google*
    (blog), November 17, 2015, https://www.michigan.gov/-/media
    /Project/Websites/mdhhs/Folder4/Folder10/Folder3/Folder110
    /Folder2/Folder210/Folder1/Folder310/Google-and-Psychological
    -Safety.pdf?rev=7786b2b9ade041e78828f839eccc8b75.

9. DaVita, "Unwavering Pursuit of a Healthier Tomorrow," n.d., accessed
    March 2023, https://www.davita.com/about.

10. Charles O'Reilly et al., "DaVita: A Community First, a Company Sec-
    ond," Stanford Graduate School of Business, 2014, https://www.gsb
    .stanford.edu/faculty-research/case-studies/davita-community-first
    -company-second.

11. Duke University, Fuqua School of Business, "DaVita CEO Kent Thiry
    on the Village," YouTube video, 3:06, 2018, https://www.youtube.com
    /watch?v=HpspRVERVR4.

12. Kim Parker, "About a Third of U.S. Workers Who Can Work from
    Home Now Do So All the Time," Pew Research Center, March 30,
    2023, https://www.pewresearch.org/short-reads/2023/03/30/about

-a-third-of-us-workers-who-can-work-from-home-do-so-all-the
-time/.

13. US Census Bureau, "The Number of People Primarily Working from Home Tripled Between 2019 and 2021," press release, September 15, 2022, https://www.census.gov/newsroom/press-releases/2022 /people-working-from-home.html.

14. Derek Thompson, "Workism Is Making Americans Miserable," *Atlantic*, February 24, 2019, https://www.theatlantic.com/ideas/archive /2019/02/religion-workism-making-americans-miserable/583441/.

15. Sahil Lavingia, "No Meetings, No Deadlines, No Full-Time Employees," *Sahil Lavingia* (blog), January 7, 2021, https://sahillavingia.com /work.

16. Rebecca Nowland, Elizabeth A. Necka, and John T. Cacioppo, "Loneliness and Social Internet Use: Pathways to Reconnection in a Digital World?," *Perspectives on Psychological Science* 13, no. 1 (2018): 70–87, https://doi.org/10.1177/1745691617713052.

17. Philippe Verduyn et al., "Do Social Network Sites Enhance or Undermine Subjective Well-Being? A Critical Review," *Social Issues and Policy Review* 11, no. 1 (January 2017): 274–302, https://doi.org/10.1111 /sipr.12033.

18. Mesfin A. Bekalu, Rachel F. McCloud, and K. Viswanath, "Association of Social Media Use with Social Well-Being, Positive Mental Health, and Self-Rated Health: Disentangling Routine Use from Emotional Connection to Use," *Health Education & Behavior* 46, no. S2 (2019): S69–80, https://doi.org/10.1177/1090198119863768.

19. Patricia McMorrow, "Mom's Approach to Breast Cancer: Keep It Positive," CaringBridge, November 19, 2021, https://www.caringbridge .org/resources/moms-positive-breast-cancer-approach/.

20. Keya Sen, Gayle Prybutok, and Victor Prybutok, "The Use of Digital Technology for Social Wellbeing Reduces Social Isolation in Older Adults: A Systematic Review," *SSM - Population Health* 17 (March 2022): 101020, https://doi.org/10.1016/j.ssmph.2021.101020.

21. Humana Foundation and Older Adults Technology Services, "Exposing the Hidden Connectivity Crisis for Older Adults," 2021, https:// agingconnected.org/wp-content/uploads/2021/05/Aging -Connected_Exposing-the-Hidden-Connectivity-Crisis-for-Older -Adults.pdf.

22. Government of India, Ministry of Electronics & Information Technology, "Digital India," n.d., accessed March 2023, https://www.digital india.gov.in/.

23. Anna Tong, "What Happens When Your Chatbot Stops Loving You Back?," Reuters, March 21, 2023, https://www.reuters.com

/technology/what-happens-when-your-ai-chatbot-stops-loving
-you-back-2023-03-18/.

24. Sangeeta Singh-Kurtz, "The Man of Your Dreams: For $300, Replika
Sells an AI Companion Who Will Never Die, Argue, or Cheat—Until
His Algorithm Is Updated," *The Cut*, March 10, 2023, https://www
.thecut.com/article/ai-artificial-intelligence-chatbot-replika
-boyfriend.html.

25. Zhang Wanqing, "The AI Girlfriend Seducing China's Lonely Men,"
Sixth Tone, December 7, 2020, https://www.sixthtone.com
/news/1006531.

26. Richie Hertzberg, "Meet the Artificially Intelligent Chatbot Trying to
Curtail Loneliness in America," *The Hill*, December 16, 2022, https://
thehill.com/changing-america/3778169-meet-the-artificially
-intelligent-chatbot-trying-to-curtail-loneliness-in-america/.

27. Laurie Clarke, "'I Learned to Love the Bot': Meet the Chatbots That
Want to Be Your Best Friend," *Guardian*, March 19, 2023, https://www
.theguardian.com/technology/2023/mar/19/i-learned-to-love-the
-bot-meet-the-chatbots-that-want-to-be-your-best-friend.

28. Rob Morris (@RobertRMorris), "We provided mental health support
to 4,000 people using GPT-3. Here's what happened," X (formerly
Twitter), January 6, 2023, https://x.com/RobertRMorris/status
/1611450197707464706?s=20.

29. Parmy Olson, "This AI Has Sparked a Budding Friendship with 2.5
Million People," *Forbes*, March 8, 2018, https://www.forbes.com/sites
/parmyolson/2018/03/08/replika-chatbot-google-machine-learning/.

Chapter 10: Flourish Together

1. Manchester Institute of Education, "The BBC Loneliness Experiment," n.d., accessed March 2023, https://www.seed.manchester
.ac.uk/education/research/impact/bbc-loneliness-experiment/.

2. Kavita Chawla et al., "Prevalence of Loneliness Amongst Older People
in High-Income Countries: A Systematic Review and Meta-Analysis,"
PLoS ONE 16, no. 7 (2021): e0255088, https://doi.org/10.1371/journal
.pone.0255088.

3. Barcelona City Council, "Barcelona contra la soledat," n.d., accessed
March 2023, https://ajuntament.barcelona.cat/dretssocials/ca
/barcelona-contra-la-soledat.

4. Robin Caruso et al., "Healthcare's Responsibility: Reduce Loneliness
and Isolation in Older Adults," *Generations Journal* (Fall 2020), https://
generations.asaging.org/healthcare-should-reduce-loneliness
-and-isolation.

5. Robin Caruso, "CareMore Health: Addressing Loneliness Leads to

Lower Rates of ED, Hospital Use," Healthcare Financial Management Association (HFMA), July 26, 2019, https://www.hfma.org /operations-management/care-process-redesign/caremore-health -addressing-loneliness-leads-to-lower-rates-of-e/.

6. Riley J. Steiner et al., "Adolescent Connectedness and Adult Health Outcomes," *Pediatrics* 144, no. 1 (July 2019): e20183766, https://doi .org/10.1542/peds.2018-3766.

7. Ryu Takizawa, Barbara Maughan, and Louise Arseneault, "Adult Health Outcomes of Childhood Bullying Victimization: Evidence from a Five-Decade Longitudinal British Birth Cohort," *American Journal of Psychiatry* 171, no. 7 (July 2014): 777–84, https://doi.org/10.1176/appi .ajp.2014.13101401.

8. Jean M. Twenge et al., "If You Can't Join Them, Beat Them: Effects of Social Exclusion on Aggressive Behavior," *Journal of Personality and Social Psychology* 81, no. 6 (2001): 1058–69, https://doi .org/10.1037/0022-3514.81.6.1058.

9. Jean M. Twenge et al., "Social Exclusion Decreases Prosocial Behavior," *Journal of Personality and Social Psychology* 92, no. 1 (2007): 56–66, https://doi.org/10.1037/0022-3514.92.1.56.

10. Ed100, "School Hours: Is There Enough Time to Learn?," n.d., accessed March 2023, https://ed100.org/lessons/schoolhours.

11. Jean M. Twenge et al., "Worldwide Increases in Adolescent Loneliness," *Journal of Adolescence* 93, no. 1 (December 2021): 257–69, https://doi.org/10.1016/j.adolescence.2021.06.006.

12. Richard Weissbourd et al., "Loneliness in America: How the Pandemic Has Deepened an Epidemic of Loneliness and What We Can Do About It," Making Caring Common Project, Harvard Graduate School of Education, February 2021, https://mcc.gse.harvard.edu/reports /loneliness-in-america.

13. Ranjini Reddy, Jean E. Rhodes, and Peter Mulhall, "The Influence of Teacher Support on Student Adjustment in the Middle School Years: A Latent Growth Curve Study," *Development and Psychopathology* 15, no. 1 (2003): 119–38, https://doi.org/10.1017 /s0954579403000075.

14. Debora L. Roorda et al., "The Influence of Affective Teacher–Student Relationships on Students' School Engagement and Achievement: A Meta-Analytic Approach," *Review of Educational Research* 81, no. 4 (2011): 493–529, https://doi.org/10.3102/0034654311421793.

15. Kathleen Moritz Rudasill et al., "A Longitudinal Study of Student–Teacher Relationship Quality, Difficult Temperament, and Risky Behavior from Childhood to Early Adolescence," *Journal of School Psychology* 48, no. 5 (October 2010): 389–412, https://doi.org/10.1016/j .jsp.2010.05.001.

16. Daniel Quin, "Longitudinal and Contextual Associations Between Teacher–Student Relationships and Student Engagement: A Systematic Review," *Review of Educational Research* 87, no. 2 (2017): 345–87, https://doi.org/10.3102/0034654316669434.

17. Nicholas C. Jacobson and Michelle G. Newman, "Perceptions of Close and Group Relationships Mediate the Relationship Between Anxiety and Depression over a Decade Later," *Depression and Anxiety* 33, no. 1 (January 2016): 66–74, https://doi.org/10.1002/da.22402.

18. Annette M. La Greca and Hannah Moore Harrison, "Adolescent Peer Relations, Friendships, and Romantic Relationships: Do They Predict Social Anxiety and Depression?," *Journal of Clinical Child & Adolescent Psychology* 34, no. 1 (2005): 49–61, https://doi.org/10.1207/s15374424jccp3401_5.

19. Paul D. Flaspohler et al., "Stand by Me: The Effects of Peer and Teacher Support in Mitigating the Impact of Bullying on Quality of Life," *Psychology in the Schools* 46, no. 7 (August 2009): 636–49, https://doi.org/10.1002/pits.20404.

20. Morning Future, "Empathy? In Denmark They're Learning It in School," April 26, 2019, https://www.morningfuture.com/en/2019/04/26/empathy-happiness-school-denmark/.

21. Inside Optimist TV, "Denmark's Education System: Where Teaching Empathy Is Part of the School Curriculum. Mariana Rudan," YouTube video, 3:37, 2019, https://www.youtube.com/watch?v=lK5fm_HLp48&list=WL&index=4.

22. Lifespan Research Foundation, "The Harvard Study of Adult Development," n.d., accessed July 2023, https://www.lifespanresearch.org/harvard-study/.

23. Jennifer Puig et al., "Predicting Adult Physical Illness from Infant Attachment: A Prospective Longitudinal Study," *Health Psychology* 32, no. 4 (2013): 409–17, https://doi.org/10.1037/a0028889.

24. S. Janet Kuramoto-Crawford, Mir M. Ali, and Holly C. Wilcox, "Parent–Child Connectedness and Long-Term Risk for Suicidal Ideation in a Nationally Representative Sample of US Adolescents," *Crisis* 38, no. 5 (2017): 309–18, https://doi.org/10.1027/0227-5910/a000439.

25. Krista Gass, Jennifer Jenkins, and Judy Dunn, "Are Sibling Relationships Protective? A Longitudinal Study," *Journal of Child Psychology and Psychiatry* 48, no. 2 (February 2007): 167–75, https://doi.org/10.1111/j.1469-7610.2006.01699.x.

26. Avidan Milevsky and Mary J. Levitt, "Sibling Support in Early Adolescence: Buffering and Compensation Across Relationships," *European Journal of Developmental Psychology* 2, no. 3 (2005): 299–320, https://doi.org/10.1080/17405620544000048.

27. Janet N. Melby et al., "Adolescent Family Experiences and Educational

Attainment During Early Adulthood," *Developmental Psychology* 44, no. 6 (2008): 1519–36, https://doi.org/10.1037/a0013352.

28. Virginia J. Noland et al., "Is Adolescent Sibling Violence a Precursor to College Dating Violence?," *American Journal of Health Behavior* 28, no. S1 (2004): S13–23, https://pubmed.ncbi.nlm.nih.gov/15055568/.

29. Robert J. Waldinger, George E. Vaillant, and E. John Orav, "Childhood Sibling Relationships as a Predictor of Major Depression in Adulthood: A 30-Year Prospective Study," *American Journal of Psychiatry* 164, no. 6 (2007): 949–54, https://doi.org/10.1176/ajp.2007.164.6.949.

30. Cari Gillen-O'Neel and Andrew Fuligni, "A Longitudinal Study of School Belonging and Academic Motivation Across High School," *Child Development* 84, no. 2 (March–April 2013): 678–92, https://doi.org/10.1111/j.1467-8624.2012.01862.x.

31. Rebecca London and Dabney Ingram, "Social Isolation in Middle School," *School Community Journal* 28, no. 1 (Spring 2018): 107–27, https://www.adi.org/journal/2018ss/LondonIngramSpring2018.pdf.

Conclusion: The Growing Social Health Movement

1. Google Trends, "'What Is Social Health' in the United States (2004–Present)," n.d., accessed September 2023, https://trends.google.com/trends/explore?date=all&geo=US&q=what%20is%20social%20health&hl=en.

2. Google Trends, "'What Is Social Health' Worldwide (2004–Present)," n.d., accessed September 2023, https://trends.google.com/trends/explore?date=all&q=what%20is%20social%20health&hl=en.

Index